M000265909

Aug

How wonderful to ~
my Auntie Marg and Un[...]
back in my life.
Much love,
Sherry

BreatheYourOMBalance
Yoga and Healing

Volume Two

Introduced by
Kelsy Timas,
Founder and CEO of Guiding Wellness Institute Inc.

Series Editors
Kitty Madden and Shana Thornton

Thorncraft Publishing
Clarksville, Tennessee

Copyright © 2018 by Thorncraft Publishing

All rights reserved.

First Edition, 2018

Published in the United States by Thorncraft Publishing.

BreatheYourOMBalance® is a registered trademark of Thorncraft Publishing.

No part of this book may be reproduced, by any means, without written permission from the author and/or Thorncraft Publishing. Requests for permission to reproduce material from this work should be sent to Thorncraft Publishing, thorncraftpublishing@gmail.com

ISBN-13: 978-0-9979687-2-9
ISBN-10: 0-9979687-2-9

Cover Design by etcetera...
Cover photo by Shana Thornton.
Cover models, Erika Wolfe and Amanda Rush,
Owners of Yoga Mat studio.

Library of Congress Control Number: 2017959537

Thorncraft Publishing
Clarksville, TN
http://www.thorncraftpublishing.com
thorncraftpublishing@gmail.com

10 9 8 7 6 5 4 3 2 1

CONTENTS

FOREWORD
By Amanda Rush

Each day, I sit on a bench in our studio sipping my coffee and watch them enter. They come in all shapes, sizes, ages, backgrounds, and ability levels. To me, they all look the same; they are souls in need of healing. As I walk through the rooms of our yoga studio, I see it happening; our yogis reach out to the new clients, speak their truth to them, and share their experiences and their stories with each other. I enter the common room and see Erika holding someone as they sob, shedding the layers that keep them bound so tight. I peek through the window into the yoga room and see one of our teachers guiding a class on how to find their breath, because so many of us have lost the ability to connect with it. Walking down the hallway, I overhear a client asking if it's normal to cry during a yoga practice. I continue on, observing, listening, and witnessing. It all comes down to one thing: Connection.

Most days the person you'll meet first when coming through our doors is Erika, the co-owner of Yoga Mat. She is our connector, our holder of space. A powerful empath, she follows intuition and goes where her heart leads. She connects on a deeper level with a human's three basic needs—to be seen, to be heard, and to be acknowledged. That is her gift that she gives to the world. These connections allow the studio to thrive. Her passion for the work we do fuels the desire of others to add their talents to the collective. They are inspired to be a part of something bigger than themselves and to make a positive impact on our community. She invites them to look within and grow their seeds of prosperity in the fertile soil she has prepared. The opportunity for this book came from such a connection. A request to post a flyer for a book signing resulted in a bond formed with the publisher, and the inspiration to collaborate on Volume 2 of the BreatheYourOMBalance book series was born.

Our studio opened in 2015, with the intention and mission to be a place where people could come to find healing on all levels. Having experienced the magic for ourselves, we have made it our life mission to provide that opportunity for everybody to heal through yoga. Believing that everything happens for a reason and trusting the process, we provide the space for miracles to happen and trust that they will. Fully supported in our mission to provide healing, a multitude of teachers and healers have appeared at our door. They all come when they are destined to be here, when their gifts and talents are made manifest to reach the people that are seeking what they can offer. Reiki masters, mystics, and teachers from the other side of the world have found their way to us to impart their wisdom. And when their mission is complete, they move on.

I witness miracles every day within our walls. Some of them happen rather quickly, while others take a bit longer. We all, in the course of our lives, have been wounded in some way, some deeper than others. Some wounds are so deep that they darken the soul and steal the light of hope that we ever may be whole again. Our life experiences, these stories of our lives, can shape who we are and influence who we become. They, in some cases, can keep us bound and act as roadblocks to the growth of the soul. They can keep us disconnected from ourselves and from others and leave us numb because it hurts too much to feel. The miracle occurs when you can transcend the circumstances of your life experience and become the witness to your story and the witness to others. Through our experience as studio owners, we have become masters of holding space, for it is in these spaces where the miracles occur. Yoga is the union of body, mind, and spirit through connection to the breath. Breath creates the space to heal. It quiets the mind, it regulates the body, and it allows for the reintegration of all the pieces of ourselves that we have lost.

Yoga finds you when you least expect. Yogis walk through our doors not knowing why they are there. They enter our space looking for something they can't quite describe. As I sit and watch, I can see it come over them almost immediately, the answers they have been searching for to the questions they haven't thought to ask. They say after entering, they can feel a calm settle over them and they feel as if they've come home. A testament to the intention we have set for the studio to be a safe space to heal is in our tagline: Be Here. Be Home. They come to us weighed down by their life experiences, closed off in fear, and running from the pain of scars long closed. The healing begins with the intention to make a change no matter the motivation. As they come through our doors, we meet them where they are and accept them for wherever that may be. When met with compassion and grace, they respond in gratitude and so begins their journey.

My role as the witness to the magic that is yoga is my greatest treasure. As Erika is the connector of the studio, I am its keeper of the energy within. My grounding presence permeates its walls as I offer my guardianship to all who enter, standing in the light, as others search for their light within. A wounding can facilitate the light of the soul to pierce the darkness and emerge stronger and brighter than before. We do not know how bright our light is until it is shadowed by the dark. I watch the struggle between darkness and light each day and witness the transformation of our yogis as they heal. Their lights grow brighter and brighter and they spread their light to others. That light is the light of hope. Hope that healing can happen. Hope that the lost find their way. Hope that those who perceive themselves as broken see the truth—that the pieces have been there all along. They just need to reconnect them.

We give these stories of hope and healing as an offering, giving gratitude to all who stand in witness to the journeys held within. The magic that happens within these pages can happen anywhere. Healing through yoga is available to all who want it. Anyone can do yoga. All you have to do is *breathe*.

BreatheYourOMBalance

Yoga and Healing
Volume Two

INTRODUCTION
By Kelsy Timas,
Founder and CEO of Guiding Wellness Institute Inc.

You may be curious about how this ancient practice called YOGA can aid in your desire to touch your toes, or maybe you are grappling with the concept of aging gracefully or living more connected and fully? Yoga is breath. But, yoga is also a practice within the breath. And when life takes your breath away, yoga is the journey of the self, through the self, back to the self. This incredible collection of poems and stories of breaking through the bulk of the body armor and peeling away the layers of pain reveals the uniqueness of this practice to each person called to the practice. What we learn first is that there is no way to do it wrong. It's what we learn on the way down that helps us when we step off the mat, and that lesson brings yoga to life and offers itself to healing.

What lies ahead as the pages grippingly unfold each reflective story of the practice is that you will discover yoga intimately, with a renewed appreciation for the raw beauty and sometimes gentle courage the mat holds for everyone called to the practice. Whether you have been to India or not, the mat, whether it is rented or bruised, calls to you *like you deserve to be here.* You plead and play with the range of sensations found just beneath the surface of the skin. Yoga, like life, can be brutal and beautiful. And as the following stories speak the language of the breath, may you be invited, affirmed, and reminded that for as long as ever, within the breath, there is always room, for all of you, here.

BreatheYourOMBalance
Yoga and Healing

Before Sunrise
Nonfiction by Brittany Howard

Begin lying on your back, knees bent with the soles of the feet grounded into the floor as the arms rest at the sides. Take a deep inhale, filling the chest and then the diaphragm. Slowly, allow the exhale to sink the body deeply into your mat, letting go of all voluntary muscle control. Listen to the breath as it flows in and out of the body making ocean wave-like sounds, softening the space between the eyebrows as if warm honey glides off the exterior of the forehead. Welcome the breath as it streams through the nostrils and pools in the space beneath the collarbones. Feel it seep through the shoulders, down the arms into the open palms of the hands, and flowing gently from the chest down the abdomen like water falling across the ribs to swirl into the pelvis. Feel the breath pour into the thighs, churn in the knees, stream down the calves and rest in the open soles of the feet. Experience the body full of the breath. Notice how you feel. Welcome anything that arises as if you had invited it.

I walk around the mirrored room, watching the rise and fall of my students' diaphragms as they breathe in and out. Behind their closed eyelids, I don't imagine what they may be trying to forget, or prepare themselves for before sunrise. Together we are here, and here we share space.

We find home on our mats like small boats on a wooden ocean. As if it is not something we do every moment of our lives, we breathe. We breathe deeply and we breathe softly. We breathe to notice how we feel. We breathe to find out what's inside. We breathe to learn how to deal with what is inside, and what is outside.

3

Together we inhale to stretch the arms to the sky. We exhale to float the arms down. We inhale the right arm up and exhale it to the left so that we can feel an opening and send breath into the expansion between each rib of the right side. With an exhale, we slowly lower the right arm down to our sides. We repeat this gesture with the left arm, to feel balanced and open through each side of the body.

We form tables with our bodies, allowing our hips to be over knees and hands beneath shoulders. Curling the toes under we press into the balls of our feet along with the mounds of the thumb, index, and pinky fingers accompanied by an inhale as we begin to lift the pelvis towards the sky. We send breath into our biceps, our deltoids, and wrists as we work to press our hips away from our hands, letting the shoulder blades melt down the back as collarbones spread wide. Here, we seek our own comfort in this demanding pose requiring full muscular body strength. We breathe in our downward facing dog.

As the sun ascends outside so do our chests, as they rise to the sky. With each inhale, we work to open and develop. Open and awaken the fascia, the connective tissues that envelop our bodies. Develop and expand our minds with understanding about the world we find ourselves in. We inhale life with the bittersweet taste of memories upon the tongue. Then before we depart, we exhale the toxins, the negative necessities of energy spent living.

We learn how to breathe in this room, before our loved ones awake to fresh cups of black coffee, before the Earth has time to absorb the night's rain, and before the day has its chance to do its worst so that when we leave here, we can still breathe out there.

The divine in me recognizes the divine in you. Namaste.

Deserving
Poetry by Jennifer Will

In the meditation hall,
I acknowledged the painted Buddha
and sat on the cushion.

The teacher said,
"Have a seat like you deserve to be here."
His teacher had said the same.

I peeked at the others who
looked comfortable, serene,
as if their knees didn't hurt.

"Have a seat like you deserve to be here."

He couldn't have meant *me...*

my mom was addicted to drugs,
I only speak one language,
I didn't get into grad school,
I'm uncomfortable in crowds,

my clothes are uncool,
I slept with strangers out of loneliness,
we were poor...

"Have a seat like you deserve to be here."

my great-uncle made moonshine
and maybe killed his brother over it,
my granddad beat his wife,

I sometimes lie about where I grew up,
I smile when I don't feel like it,
I eat meat,

I've never been to India,
I've never been to Europe,
I really couldn't afford this retreat
or the last one.

They know I'm not one of them.

"Have a seat like you deserve to be here."

The tears, they broke the dam of my eyes,
rained over my cheeks.
My knees, they hurt,
so I got up and sat in a chair.

The Magic of Restorative Yoga
Nonfiction by Sherry Ulansky

Yoga is supposed to be good for you, right? That's what I'd been told, so I thought I would give it a try.

I was grappling with the concept of aging gracefully in a culture that values youth over living youthfully. When I looked in the mirror, I wasn't pleased with the effect fifty years of gravity was having on my body. Was I destined to never feel beautiful again because of wrinkles, grey hair, menopausal hot flashes, and a larger waistline than I had in my twenties?

At forty-five, the disks in my cervical spine herniated. The cumulative impact of three car accidents in my twenties and thirties had finally caught up with me. Then at forty-seven, I started a job facilitating on-line courses that required six to eight hours of computer work per day, further compounding the physical problems. I wasn't relishing the thought of spending the rest of my life in constant pain, so I started to investigate alternatives to surgery and pain-killers. Yoga was part of that search.

I gave several different kinds a try. At hatha, I couldn't touch the floor in a forward bend, my knees wouldn't touch the ground in the lotus position, and I pulled a groin muscle trying the warrior pose. My hips were too tight for that. My focus at kundalini was to avoid passing out doing the breath work at a pace so fast I hyperventilated in seconds. No thanks.

I moved onto hot yoga next. I love the heath care practitioner who suggested it, but he's never had the pleasure of a menopausal hot flash. I'd feel the internal furnace in my belly firing up in the middle of class, my sweat production would quadruple instantaneously, and I'd be back to focusing on not passing out. Next class, please.

Flow and power flow made me question my judgment on the whole yoga pursuit. I was continually two poses behind. The instructor was up, I'm down; the instructor is forward, I'm still looking at the back of the room. All I heard was "Pick it up ladies. Burn those calories." Burn those calories!? I was trying to relax, not attend a cardio class.

I'm a Type A person. I didn't need to attend a Type A yoga class that revved me up rather than relaxed me.

A year or so into the pursuit of the perfect yoga practice, I observed a disheartening pattern. I'd have a major neck and back flare-up every three or four months, beginning with a headache that would not go away, followed by that telltale twinge in my neck that meant my cervical spine was inflamed which ultimately led to weeks of excruciating pain. Frustrated beyond words, I was ready to give up. Fortunately, an act of providence was about to change my course.

In 2013, I received a Christmas gift from my boss for a "Do Less" Restorative Yoga Retreat. I walked into the dinner hall and met Tim. At six feet, four inches tall, he had the body of a long-distance runner, but carried himself like a professional dancer; his movements graceful and fluid.

"Welcome to a weekend of doing less," he said.

Okay, I could get into that.

Doing Less. I spent three glorious days enveloped in a fleece blanket to maximize the heat from a biomat beneath me. Every pose supported by blocks, straps, and bolsters; I did not miss hyperventilating, profuse sweating, and being two poses behind. Legs supported by bolsters in a two-knee twist, a lavender pillow across my eyes, I'd wait for Tim to give me a Thai head massage. It was an entire weekend of absolute bliss.

I'd found a practice that worked for my body and left me feeling relaxed, so I purchased private restorative sessions. Was it expensive? Yes. But, how much did I value a pain-free body?

I blocked off an hour-and-a-half on Thursdays and committed to showing up at Tim's studio every week. And so began my journey of healing.

I always considered myself to be diligent at making time and space to look after myself. I went for massages, took dancing lessons, meditated, swam, went for long walks in the forest with friends, and enjoyed cultural events. I believed that all the fun things I filled my life with in order to unwind were successfully accomplishing that purpose. As the weeks unfolded on the floor of Tim's studio, I was to discover differently.

Restorative yoga is slow. My Type A brain couldn't quite figure out how anything that didn't require a lot of work was going to benefit my body. "No pain, no gain," right? Slowly, I started to discover that those long, supported poses were allowing my body to fully engage and soften. The areas that held all my tension or were injured began to realign. Ever so gently, the magic of restorative yoga started to happen.

At first, I noticed small, subtle changes. I got bendier. I began picking up socks from the floor without bending my knees, and those knees would actually touch the floor when I sat cross-legged. That led to bigger stuff; kayaking without having the discs in my neck complain. The cervical spine flare-ups pretty much disappeared.

One day was remarkable. Amid numerous props, cocooned in a fleece blanket and biomats, I had my nirvana moment, experiencing that level of stillness and tranquility that had eluded me with other yoga styles.

No more racing. There I was, lying on the floor crying because my bullet train of a nervous system had finally slowed down. No, not just slowed down, come to a halt.

That moment was the beginning of an entirely different way to live my life. Tim and I spent hours talking about his philosophy of how "Doing less at the right time allows you to do more at the appropriate time." Unwinding is no longer an exercise of mental or physical distraction.

Having embodied the experience of "Doing Less", I've become much more protective of the time needed to achieve that. My yoga mat, bolsters, and blankets have become my sanctuary from an active life—a haven of regeneration.

I accomplished my quest for a yoga practice that has helped me cope with the challenges of aging. As I approach my sixties, I recognize that it has given me much more. Those moments of quiet on my mat provide me with the opportunity to re-evaluate how I engage in a productive and active life, while maintaining an internal calm more consistently. I treasure the coherence of body, mind, and spirit it affords.

"Beauty" is no longer defined by an absence of wrinkles, grey hair, or sagging body parts. Without the constant internal chatter and raciness, I'm able to access and embrace the wisdom and grace that come with those wrinkles, grey hair, and sagging parts. That's what makes me beautiful!

So yes, yoga is good for you, especially when you find the right kind!

Yoga Mat
Poetry by Yvette Huber

Fly Paper: Sticking hands into the mat in a clumsy
Downward Dog; anxious and trapped.

Microscope Slide: Feeling exposed in this awkward position;
Yet everyone else is focused on their *drishti*.

Raft: Adrift on waves of uncertainty;
Dive into the deep, resurface in Upward Dog.

Canvas: Form and contour emerge in Warrior stance;
Light and shadows interplay.

Sponge: Sweat drips off extended limbs;
Mat absorbs what is released.

Mirror: Gazing down from Airplane Pose;
What is reflected back?

Flower Bed: Grounding down, digging in;
               Seed must break for growth to occur.

Coffin: Boxed in Corpse Pose;
               Waiting to arise from *Savasana*.

Door Mat: Step across the threshold;
               Anticipating the next leg of the journey.

Band Aid: Mat rips off the floor;
               The healing practice continues.

Dialects of Yoga
Nonfiction by Ericka Suhl

What kind of foreign language is this? I have a certain dialect of movement that does not sound at all like these wide, balanced stances. Try as I might to pronounce the poses correctly, the idea of spreading my toes has to start with the realization that I have toes in the first place. These toes? The toes I have stuffed into pointed shoes with pointed heels all these years? Balance used to mean staying afloat in the world atop ankle-straining spindles, and now I have to learn how to fix my feet broadly and directly upon—no—*into* the earth. Yoga's language of motion demands subtle intonation. When my body stands in mountain pose, I step into the earth.

"Listen to your body."

When it is screaming? Isn't that the norm? When I hit the stairs at work with my bag filled with books, papers, files and calendars, and my left knee sings out a dying call, full of fire, I listen. I listen because the pain ripples out of my body, like sound waves, beyond the borders of flesh. Why, then, is it so hard for me to imagine that my energy can flow into the ground, from my heart, through my legs, and out of my long-ignored toes?

"Reach."

Now I can hear my heart beat, and feel my face flush with blood and heat. At first, warrior pose is a simple script. I stretch my arms into the air, and there is nothing above or below me. My legs are wide beneath my arms, and my chest is open. And then my mind begins to drift. I carry anxieties around in a way that makes me top-heavy, like my head weighs a thousand pounds.

"Focus on your breathing."

I am. I'm breathing hard. It's impossible to ignore. The "nothing" that I hold my arms out into feels exponentially heavy once it is mixed up with time. My body hums in a low register of panic, as if, at any moment, all my joints will sound off in a chorus of burning pain. The energy I send out into the universe is tired, weakened, and broken. I am scared. This is not my language. This is not my home. I am thrusting my body out, in all directions, and the weight of this world challenges every inch of my boundaries. I'm about to be crushed like an aluminum can.

"Quiet your mind."

I will. I am. Where am I? Probably in the dark, with light coming in through the windows of the studio, and there are other women here with their own pressures upon them, and—whoa! Did you see her? Did you see what she did with her leg during tree pose? I've never even seen a *tree* do that. She looks like she stepped right out of the cover of *Yoga Journal.* I'll never be able to do that. In a million years of several reincarnations, I'll still fold as awkwardly as the Tin Man. My body speaks this language coarsely, all lumps and drama. I can't. I can't. I just can't.

***

Shirley is a petite woman with white hair and clear blue eyes. Though I would never say it to her face, in my mind I call her "Big Shirl." When she teaches her relaxation classes, her radiance fills the room, overwhelming me with the perception that she is much larger than her frame. However, this radiance is not a great and terrible thing, so perhaps "overwhelming" isn't the right word. There is too much peace and calm in the light she carries, and I can't find the word that describes something that at once is a force and its opposite. My only associations with force have had to do with breaking and unmaking, not healing.

The whole idea behind her class could be told as a joke. I drive to the studio, pay the fee, and then rest with all my might, but it is something that I need much guidance with. Following strict orders from my therapist that I find some way to relax, I found Shirley's class listed online, and looked at it as a last-ditch effort to find true restoration in the language of yoga. I trust my therapist, who is tasked with treating me for the kind of depression that comes with constant, incurable illness. I have Crohns disease, a condition that requires steadfast management to remain in remission. Otherwise, the painful, life-altering symptoms can generate depression which exacerbates the gut-held inflammation due to stress and anxiety which sets off more pronounced and painful symptoms, heightening the intensity of the depression, and so it goes and so it goes in an endless cycle. Under these circumstances, finding help to relax is, for me, serious business.

Shirley starts her sessions with a warm smile and a few blood pumping stances, but then we're soon on the floor with cushions and covers. The whole class is geared toward relaxation, and while our poses are deliberate, they are the poses of children asleep. Still, Shirley asks us to breathe into our poses, much like every other instructor I've had, calling attention to the fact that achieving deep relaxation and rest can be just as difficult as mastering inversion or balance poses. With the cushions and blankets positioned under me, just so, I feel the tension that I need to release bubble outward from spaces deep within my body. I am tender about my gut, spending most of my life protecting it with a pronounced slouch. Shirley walks through her students as we sit and breathe, and she provides a tiny touch in the middle of my back. It is the slightest adjustment needed to open my chest a little more, letting in a little more air, taking a little more pressure off my lower back, my shoulders, and my neck. One tiny movement melts away a glacier's worth of slow-creeping tension.

There are times that, during the side poses on the floor, I feel like I might cry. It is a curious dialect that I never would have thought existed in yoga. Perhaps, whatever is in me that is melting and breaking apart into something like tears is the word I am looking for that combines the connotations of peace and disruption. It is a word that only exists in yoga and can only be said with the body, and the result of this word's resonance throughout that body is joyful surrender. Perhaps that awareness has been missing all these years while I've struggled as a yoga novice. It is possible to be at once broken and mended. I leave Shirley's classes wondering just how I'll react to more aggressive yoga flow sessions, and if I need anything more than her gentle reminders to open up a little bit more, a tiny bit more.

***

Alex is at the studio today and I'm glad to see her because strange things have been happening. She warned me after our last session that I might feel emotional or insecure, and I wondered, "Some difference. I always feel emotional and insecure."

Alex is a young woman with bright, hazel eyes and long, dark hair. The energy in her face is focused and friendly. It's as if her mind doesn't stay guarded within her head. She thinks in a focused radiance that ranges out, always forward, from her face at least seven feet or hours or days in front of her. Her hair and hands move as if picked up by the wind of her own forward energy. Standing in the way of her energy is always more welcoming than I imagine, and so I feel like I can tell her things that make me feel a little crazy.

She directed our class through a series of hip openers a day or two before, and of course I've been feeling insecure because that never goes away. But something very strange is happening.

"I'm having memories that I haven't had in many years. Memories from long ago. And they're nice memories. When I see something that would normally make me feel insecure, I'm suddenly reminded of something good."

Alex thinks about what I've said, way out of her head, around mine, bouncing her thoughts off the walls when she says, "We keep a lot of things in our hips. When you open them up, all that stuff gets released."

I've heard that said before, never imagining what kind of "stuff" my instructors could be talking about. No one had specifically said that I would find myself anxious about driving home along I-65 and I-24 late at night after Christmas shopping in Nashville. No one said that I would watch the headlights and brake lights and street lights go by. No one promised that these lights would fill me with a tremendous amount of peace and joy because I would feel, absolutely, like I was back in Seattle, where I was young, where I had friends, before the wars and the sicknesses and the surgeries that would come. No one said, "The lights will at once be Nashville after the scars and Seattle before them, with all the sunsets of Elliott Bay, the Sound stretching up to Canada, and the lights of downtown whizzing by as you drive, once again, along the viaduct, to your own home that you made out of your hopes and dreams." No one warned me that I would enjoy feeling the past again; I could think about those things and live briefly within them again, without pain or loneliness.

Alex looks away from her thoughts back to me, meets my eyes, and says, "It is different for everyone."

***

It's moving day for some friends who are getting married soon. I'm hauling boxes of their shoes, spices, and books up the narrow steps of their new home in South Nashville, and I feel my strength reach out of the ground, through my core, into my own tensile nature, like the giant tree in their yard that sways firmly in its space. My legs and arms work in concert to the beat of each step, and my lungs are filled with cool, fall air. It's almost Christmas again, and I've been going to the yoga studio for nearly a year, finding new methods of yoga practice that activate parts of my body and soul I never knew existed before taking those first simultaneous reaches into spaces inside and spaces outside. While I help my friends move into their first home together, my body speaks its own easy and confident dialect. I feel no pain.

I was anxious about helping them move. It's that thing most people do only for those they really care about, and it is done with the expectation that many things will still be left unpacked, the best laid plans of truck pick-ups and drop-offs will fail, and everyone will be miserable. It will also rain. I was particularly sensitive about my gut. Lifting takes a good, solid core, and my gut is diseased. For six weeks, lightning bolts of panic had been shooting through my core at random in an unrelenting, stagnant storm of anxiety. My husband is a soldier, and he was off to war again. We prepared, as a family, and we spent our last moments together having fun as a family. My son experienced his summer break out of a suitcase as we traveled far and wide before our year-long separation. I met my husband in 2002, and we have spent our entire married lives under the shadow of continuous war, so I knew the patterns to come. It would take him a while, but he would arrive in Afghanistan, get established, and within two weeks I would get my first phone call from him. When it came, I was driving. He asked me to pull the car over. He told me that he wanted a divorce. I have not heard his voice since.

He was worried that this change would trigger a Crohns attack, and he urged me to take care of myself. He told me not to hurt myself. He told me that my son needed me. Then, he said nothing at all. My yoga practice has been rooted in opening up the unexplored, and the feelings that surged through me, once I knew my marriage had to end, were unlike anything my body had spoken before. There are no words for the feelings. They continue to rattle through me as electricity, fire, nonsense. I have to completely reshape all aspects of my future, and I've never felt more vulnerable, and yet...

"Breathe."

And yet, I am stepping into the earth, with boxes of my friends' things firmly balanced in my arms, practicing the back and forth, reaching and lifting movements that I'll make with my own things in a few months as I find a new place to live with my son. He's here too, watching me move confidently with the strange swells of the bumpy front yard, and he is carrying what a little boy can while I guide him. We glide through the chaotic and exhausted movements of several people who came to help, all lifting up, asking where, and placing carefully, one object at a time. We are all collectively there to help. They all know what I'm going through, and they're all talking about how we will all see each other again when it's time to pick me up and put me somewhere new.

***

I thought my first session of yoga Nidra would go a lot like Shirley's class. It was supposed to offer intense healing while I lay on the ground completely relaxed. The Nidra classes are still held in the evenings, after the pulse of the day has slowed. That first night, I found the light blue studio walls warmed by the orange glow of candlelight. There were more blankets and towels laid out than in any other practice, and Linda, my Nidra guide, appeared softly into that space, offering me essential oils. Linda was a little hard to believe at first, because her face, body, and gestures spoke love. It wasn't weird, because I felt completely at ease around her, but it certainly didn't represent the kind of energy I typically encountered. I have only felt similar in the presence of experienced nurses who are calm and steady about providing comfort and ending pain. That level of care is, in fact, exactly what Linda provides in her yoga practice. Nidra is a practice that aims its healing power at the deepest tears and fractures, and Linda's voice was my first guide into that awareness.

I followed her calm and soothing suggestions to focus on my breath while remaining conscious of the sounds all around me, in the room and outside of it. Her voice acted as a hand to hold through a dark cave, and she asked me to be aware of how cold my toes and fingers had grown and how warm my shoulders and hips felt as they connected to the ground. My awareness moved across my body until the heaviness of sleep took my body without taking my consciousness with it. When it was time to look into memories of joy, and memories of stress, I could calmly observe myself in those memories instead of shivering terrified in the clash and bang of a subconscious nightmare. I was aware, awake, and at rest. When the memory of watching the golden koi at the zoo with my son came to me, the koi swam smoothly out of the dark and they brought with them a feeling of complete peace. During the stressful memory, I was back in the hospital, eight Christmases ago, when I was fighting for my life after emergency surgery brought on by Crohns complications. I could smell the oxygen from my mask and taste the saline from my IV, as if I was there again, but the terror was gone. I moved into the memory and out of it again, feeling the moment with the pain turned off. The koi were swimming all around. I was at peace.

Yoga Nidra became my favorite practice, and while I'm happy to let any of the instructors guide me through, I am still partial to Linda's voice and go on the best internal journeys with her. During one journey through myself, I fixed upon the metaphor of a Chinese snake. I had been having a little fun with Chinese astrology earlier that day, but the fun was tempered with tension because even then it was clear that my husband was pulling away. That night during my Nidra practice, I imagined a giant, red snake, drawn like a Chinese caricature, living in my gut, tangled throughout it. The more I relaxed into the practice, the more the snake slithered and moved. The metaphor became a feeling, a tingling that I could follow with my mind, and at the most intensive moment of the session, the snake raced its way up my spine and out of the top of my head into God knows where. When Linda checked in on me after the session, all I could say for it was, "It was great. Things got pretty weird." During Nidra, while I glide easily into memories of my first roller skates on Christmas morning, I can feel locked-up, painful memories uncoiling, agitated and ready for a new home somewhere else. They burst out of the top of my head, de-fanged, de-venomed.

***

How did I wind up here? I was all set to stick with my normal morning practice in the big, blue room, and then something called me into this little sunburnt room with only three other people, piercing sunshine, and insufferable heat. Erika, the studio's owner, sets up her popular class in the largest room where she has been helping me with my body's dialect, finding ways to help me open up my joints, my back, like long vowels sounded out into an "om" of infinite breath. There is always more space between my shoulders, along my ribs, locked within my hips, and down deep in the bottom of my lungs. My throat burned like it was on fire during my first practices so badly that I felt like I was slowly choking. I would pull at my neck to try to make space for the air. It's been months since I've felt like that. Now the air moves through me unbound and clean. I still cannot put my foot behind my head, but I finally understand that I don't need to in order to do yoga "right." The act of *trying* to put my foot behind my head is all the movement I need to find new spaces. Let me clarify that "trying" may be seen as a calm moment of holding my foot in my hand for a few breaths while I look at my toenails and consider what color to paint them next. It's my practice. I've been more disciplined about showing up for sessions because I know I'll feel better as soon as my butt hits the mat. I was ready to hear Erika's voice, and then Cali walked into a small room I never paid attention to before, full of sun, and I wanted to be in there instead. Something unseen practically pushed me into this little space, and here I am.

Cali has a bright face with strong features and an ever-changing smile that waxes and wanes as she thinks through the movements of her practice, and hers is a practice of dragons and warriors.

"The Dragon uncurls her tail."

Cali teaches Yang yoga, and I have been shifting and sliding all over the floor, tapping the walls for balance, and sweating all over my body. I have pulled in Chi and pushed out warrior poses. What's crazy is, I'm hanging with this. I'm okay. All the other ladies have carried me to this moment. Erika's beloved spaces are open just enough. Linda and Alex uncoil the physical and emotional tension locked in my hips *just enough*. Shirley's adjustments help me to balance *just enough*. Now Cali is helping me breathe into warrior stances that I'm not doing in any other dialect but my very own, and it's *just enough*.

"The Dragon spreads her wings."

I can feel the wobble while I balance and hear Alex's voice in my head call out, "The wobble is good! It means you're doing it right. If you knock over your neighbor, you get a free pizza." I look over at my mat-mates, and we're all sweating and struggling, and getting through this rigorous flow together. I brought a divorce and Crohns disease into this little studio room, and no one has time to let that fact slow them down. They have their own things locked in their own joints that they're trying to break open for a little more space. Their bodies speak their own dialects, and we all understand each other. We are on our last round of Dragon flows, and I find myself holding the poses a little longer, relishing the sweat and instability. We are dancing up to our limitations and challenging them together. In a few breaths we will fall to our mats laughing. Once we catch our breath, we'll resolve to make up dragon names for ourselves. When Cali bows her final "Namaste," her smile will be radiant. But first, we have one last pose.

"The Dragon flies."

The Practice of Sharing Your Practice
Nonfiction by Nikki Martin

I've struggled with the debate that a yoga practice is private, not to be shared, especially as someone who shares it through social media and yet wants deeply to protect the practice. I can't profess to know what's right but I can tell you what I've come to believe.

Share the hell out of your yoga practice. When you learn on your mat to pause before you react, give that same pause to others and shift how they move on from their interactions with you. As you build kindness, compassion, and love for yourself, take that softer version out into the world so that other people might see it and soften a little towards themselves, and each other. When you learn to move through your practice with devotion and delight, share that, that reminder of the utter miracle of all this great big messy, painful, beautiful whole of our human existence.

Share the joy and don't hide the sorrow. Share how you let yourself stumble and fall, and then get back up again with grace and humility, or maybe something else, and yet still you press on. Share that sense of being content with where you are, paired with that willingness to keep the fire burning that takes you further than you'd ever dared to dream. Share it all.

Good, bad, and every damn thing in-between. Give it away until there is nothing left but space to fill up again with whatever you choose. This is not a practice of accumulation—of things kept for ourselves. We are in the practice of being better so we can take that out into the world. We are in the practice of building strong, beautiful, and authentic relationships with ourselves so that we can connect with each other in a deeper and more honest way. Really connect.

This is a practice of love. Love—a thing that can never be possessed only cultivated, discovered, remembered, and given so that it can build and grow, this drawing back and in before pouring out again, the beginning of a wave so powerful nothing can truly escape its crashing.

Do I know what's right? No. But my heart whispers all this to me when I'm wandering in the dark, and so I listen, and I share, and I try over and over again to be the person my heart thinks I can be.

So here's to you. All you sharers, lovers, dreamers, artists, wordsmiths, adventurers, yoga pose capturers, underwear yogis, nude yogis, head-to-toe covered yogis, yogis without labels, poets, teachers, students, believers, love warriors, all of you. Keep sharing. Keep reminding each other and me that there's a purpose to it all.

One Practice at a Time
Nonfiction by Sophia Winters

I read all the quotes....

"...sometimes all you need is twenty seconds of insane courage. (...) And I promise you, something great will come of it."—Benjamin Mee from *We Bought a Zoo.*

"And suddenly you know—it's time to start something new and trust the magic of new beginnings."—Meister Eckhart

"You can't start the next chapter of your life if you keep re-reading the last one."—Anonymous

"Making a big life change is pretty scary. But, know what's even scarier? Regret."—Zig Zigler

...and the list continues.

So, I did it. I followed my dream.

And, I shattered into a thousand tiny pieces.

While there may be quotes for heartbreak, there are truly no words for the darkness. No tape, no glue, just a thousand tiny pieces of a lost dream. Every time I attempted to pick up the pieces, I cut myself on the shattered glass.

To say, "Time heals all wounds" implies there is an end, a point in which there will be repair or closure. I can't see that. I am forever changed. It lingers just below the surface. I will say that time lessens the intensity, takes away the rawness, and allows us to survive. We remain in a state of recovery, able to choose another plan, whether it's B, C, D,...A is no longer an option.

When I hit this low point in my life, a few people offered advice: try some meds for a little while, see a therapist, write in a journal, practice yoga and meditation. All of the suggestions assumed I wanted to get better and to move on with my life. Yet, the darkness—it is so very dark. I couldn't see my hand in front of my face. There seemed to be an endless, overwhelming succession of hopeless days. Where is the path, once the dream has disappeared?

Finally, I did see a therapist. She wanted to go back and to discuss the foundation of my lost dream. Perhaps she hoped to help me build a new, better dream. I didn't return to find out. I spent my days in tears, crying an endless river of emotion. I couldn't shake it, couldn't snap out of it. There are days, weeks, and events that I can't recall. Darkness, alcohol, sleep—those are the things I remember.

Eventually, after years, not days or weeks, I discovered my own yoga practice. The darkness has not disappeared. It stays with me, but the person I am on the mat is able to fight the demons. My yoga journey has brought gratitude, beauty, grace, and belief back into my life. Peace is slowly building in my heart. I am picking up the pieces one practice at a time.

There's another popular quote, by Pema Chodron, "Nothing ever goes away until it teaches us what we need to know." The lost dream and ensuing darkness continue to teach me that happiness is on the inside. It also calls me to reach out and share my thoughts on depression and yoga and meditation.

Here's what I wish my therapist had said, "This is a seven-day guide to surviving this week. There is no quick fix, no easy solution. We all handle grief differently. Yes, you are grieving. Something very special and important to you has been taken away and there is no going back. I know today, it doesn't seem like you can survive this, but I promise, you can. You just need to hold on while you do. I'll be waiting for you here next Tuesday."

Week 1

Day 1 – Take a shower, and change your pajamas. Attend to your most basic needs. Put a cold, wet washcloth over your face to help with the headache and swollen eyes. Sleep.

Day 2 – Grieve for your loss. Repeat Day 1.

Day 3 – Find your favorite blanket or towel. Repeat Day 1.

Day 4 – Bring your favorite blanket or towel into another room. Place it on the floor and practice child's pose. Close your eyes and count to sixty. Stay in this fetal-like position as long as it feels comfortable. Rise slowly and try to eat a little something—whatever you can hold down. Get more sleep and remember your most basic self-care needs.

Day 5 – Return to child's pose today on your favorite blanket or towel. Again count to sixty. When you're ready, stretch out on your stomach. Place your forehead on the blanket/towel and your arms somewhere that feels comfortable. Count to sixty. Stay here until you're ready to return to child's pose. Rise slowly and change your sheets.

Day 6 – Start in child's pose again today. Count to sixty. Then stretch out on your stomach. Place your forehead on the blanket/towel and your arms above your head. Slowly lift your left arm and right leg. Count to ten. Change to your right arm and left leg. Count to ten. As your energy allows, repeat. Return to child's pose. Rise slowly and grab a light snack.

Day 7 – Yes, return to child's pose for sixty seconds. Then, enjoy a nice stretch onto your stomach. Place your hands under your forehead and slide your left leg to a ninety-degree angle. Count to sixty and repeat with your right leg. Return to child's pose. Rise slowly. Go to your closet and take out your favorite casual outfit. You'll need this for your appointment with the therapist tomorrow. It's time for another seven-day survival guide.

So begins the most basic foundation of a yoga practice. Going to a yoga class can be intimidating, especially in those dark days of depression. I didn't want to see anyone, talk to anyone, or do anything. Today, I like the quiet of being on my mat alone, able to flow through the poses of my choosing. I consider it a moving meditation. Once I made the commitment to practice daily, whether that is fifteen minutes or more than an hour, it has become a part of my life, of who I am. It has changed how I see myself, and more than anything, I believe again.

Being on the mat is both a mental and physical experience. How can stretching bring about such a change? As the quote by Judith Hanson

Lasater goes, "It's not about touching your toes. It's about what you learn on the way down." It's about looking for your inner self, for taking the time to slow down, to be in the moment, to focus all of your strength and energy on holding a pose, and for reaching deep into yourself to find that inner peace.

It's palpable. I feel it, just as I surrender and then release from the asana. In that moment of surrender, I can feel the light and warmth radiating through the cracks and crevices of the shattered heart I've been slowly putting back together—one practice at a time.

"Courage does not always roar. Sometimes courage is the quiet voice at the end of the day saying, 'I will try again tomorrow.'"—Mary Anne Radmacher, from the book, *Courage Does Not Always Roar: Ordinary Women with Extraordinary Courage*

Please
Poetry by E.W. Dziadon III

I walked aboard the crowded plane.
The passengers all bound east.
I sensed, and then saw a Punjabi woman
stifling her grief. I lingered
for a moment. Her voice was soft and meek.
She was in America when her husband met eternal sleep.
Her heaving sobs began to grow
And mine along with hers.
"Give me your pain. Give me your woes.
I'm strong enough for both."
Projecting these thoughts towards her mind and hoping
she would catch a glimpse
of how much gentler life could be
if she could utilize my gift.

Firelight
Haiku by Laura Hurn

A firefly sun dance.
Sun rays burn glittery wings.
Damaged wings soar anon.

A Yoga Journey
Nonfiction by April McDunn

Six years ago, I had never done a downward facing dog. I didn't even own a yoga mat. But six years ago, without my knowing, my yoga journey began.

August 13, 2011

It was a slow night at the restaurant where I was working and having been on a double shift, I got cut first to go home. At 9:02 p.m., I sent a text to my then boyfriend, now husband, Will, that I was off work. He sent a reply at 9:03 p.m., and I didn't see it until after. As I was walking to my car, I was grabbed from behind with a knife held to my throat. I was told to do everything this person said and I wouldn't be hurt. Two and a half hours later, I called Will in a panic, "I was just raped."

When I said that, it wasn't real. It wasn't real when I was at the police station, when I was driven to the hospital, when the detective came to my home so I could pick a man from a line up. It wasn't real. It wasn't real until I sat alone with these thoughts in my head and really began to think of what had happened. The trauma I had endured. This was real; this terrible thing was real. Meeting with attorneys, police officers, victims' rights advocates, doctors, this became my life. Attorneys came to my work, and police were offered to escort me to and from my job. I was told not to go anywhere alone. Every day, I woke up with this dark feeling surrounding me.

I met with advocates. I called a few hotlines. I saw therapist after therapist. Then, I got tired. I got tired of talking about it because it consumed me. When I was having a good day, I'd have a flashback or something I saw would make me think of this traumatic experience. When I was sleeping, I had the most terrible dreams and would relive every detail. And then I had to talk about it when I didn't want to in my therapy sessions. So, I started to ignore it and refused to talk about it. That was the worst decision I had ever made.

June 2012 - December 2013

My husband and I moved to Tennessee where he was stationed with the Army. We got our first home, and we explored our new town finding new places to visit and hang out. Then, my husband deployed in September, and I decided to stay in our new home. I was alone a lot. I had friends, but they had husbands and families who were at home. During this time alone, I sunk into a very dark place. I would go to work, come straight home, and lock myself in the house. While cooking dinner, I would be out of butter and need it for a recipe. I wouldn't go out to get butter; instead, I would stop making dinner or make something else. On weekends, I woke up early to do my grocery shopping and any other errands, then went straight home and slept the rest of the day away. For nine months, this was my life.

When my husband came home, I was different. I didn't even know who I was or what I even wanted in life anymore. I wasn't happy with who I had let myself become. I defined myself and my life by what had happened to me. I was pushing my family and friends away, my biggest and best support system. I had to do something, so I went back to a therapist.

December 2013 – May 2016

This seemed to help for a bit and then I started to dread going. I felt like I had talked it over so much that I kept saying I felt the same way over and over. I still looked behind me in stores. I struggled going out to dinner with friends because it'd be dark when I'd get home. I was still scared.

Then, a friend invited me to a yoga class. I was so excited! I'd always wanted to get into a yoga class and learn all those awesome poses I saw online. I didn't know at the time it was so much more than cool poses.

My first class was amazing. I didn't know half of what I was doing, but I can tell you I was hooked from that day. I realized as I was lying in savasana that I hadn't thought about anything. It had been years since my mind was quiet. I sunk onto my mat, feeling light and free. I had never felt better.

Each practice after the first, I gave my all on my mat. I practiced on my good days and walked away feeling amazing. I practiced on my bad days and got off my mat proud of myself for pushing through the day and showing up on my mat.

I started to come back to myself. I wasn't going to be the same person I was before, but I knew I could rediscover pieces of myself that I loved before and could love again. With positive affirmations, setting motivating intentions, and taking the time for self-care and love, I started to change.

May 2016 – August 2016

In May of 2016, one of my fellow classmates at my then-current studio told me to try out a new studio called Yoga Mat. She said they offered a wider variety of classes (I was strictly doing Hot 26 and vinyasa classes for the past two-and-a-half years) and the people at the new studio were home, which was a foreign way to put it in my mind, as I had come from a studio that was very business oriented. I had gotten close with a few of the teachers but they were there to teach the class they had put together and then go home. So, Yoga Mat was a 180-degree different type of studio. The first time I went to Yoga Mat, I was greeted with a huge hug by a glowing woman who just radiated love. Little did I know, this woman would help me further my yoga in a way that I hadn't even known it could grow.

I practiced at Yoga Mat regularly as Will, my husband, was away for trainings every other month. My practice continued to give me the "free-time" my mind needed. I started to grow very close to some of my classmates and even closer to that glowing woman, Erika, as well as Amanda and Alex. They became my family. We had very funny moments together, and then could turn around and have the most serious, life-changing conversations. It was so great to have them as my family and support while Will was away. Then one day, Erika came up to me and said that I should look into the Yoga Teacher Training they were hosting at Yoga Mat with Guiding Wellness coming up in February 2017. She said that she could see me doing very well in the program and that I'd enjoy learning more about yoga other than the postures.

32

I went to class and didn't think anything of it until I got home later and did some reading on the Guiding Wellness website. I got excited just reading over the material and knew I'd thoroughly enjoy it, but couldn't bring myself to say "yes" to it. I had all sorts of "why nots" running through my head. I didn't know if we'd be in Tennessee the whole time for me to complete the course. I thought, *What are people going to say when I tell them I'm going to become a yoga instructor?* And the biggest one, *I can't do this for myself. What did I do to deserve this opportunity?* So, I tucked it away in the, "I'd love to, but can't convince myself I deserve this" file.

Then, Alex caught me. I was checking out the training flyer they had hung up all over the studio one day before class. She said, "I know class is about to start and I want to talk to you more about this after, but take this training, April." I went to class and this time, I couldn't stop thinking about that training. I sat down with Alex after our class and she told me what she had been through in her life and how pivotal an experience her teacher training had been. That really got me thinking. *What if, after all this time of holding onto what happened to me, it was time for me to start taking myself back? What if I AM worth this? Why can't I do this?* I made the decision, without even telling anyone that I was signing up for the program. I hit submit on the email. I hadn't been more excited about anything as I had sending that email in a very long time.

August 2016 – February 23, 2017

This period was a really fun one. I started telling people about my upcoming training, with no shame and all the excitement, probably going into so much detail people didn't care to hear but I wanted to share. Then, my application came for financial assistance, and the acceptance of this assistance. I had my phone interview with Guiding Wellness and hadn't been so nervous for anything as I had then. The phone interview went well in my opinion, and it was the time to just wait and see if I'd be one of the lucky ones to get a slot. Next, one of the best days arrived. The day I was just scrolling through my emails and saw my Welcome Packet from Guiding Wellness into the 200 Hour Therapeutic Yoga Teacher Training for 2017! I was over the moon and even more excited than I thought I could be. It was my time to shine!

February 24, 2017

It was a Friday, and I couldn't think of a single thing all day other than getting to class that night. I was beyond ready. I met all my classmates, nervous and too scared to talk to anyone even though we'd be spending more than 200 hours together over the next nine months. Then, we had our open share circle. This was an experience. As each person told their story, I saw that all these people have pieces of me in them, and I have their pieces in me. That's the moment I knew that I was exactly where I needed to be.

February 24, 2017 – Present Day

Almost four years later, my practice continues to change me. I grow with each breath. I become stronger with each inhale and let go of a past I can't change with each exhale. Things are bad, then worse, and then they start to get better. I am not defined by the things that happened to me. I am defined by the things I chose to be. I am strong. I am happy. I am a warrior. All because of this beautiful practice that is yoga.

All of this has been shown to me time and time again during my experience in this teacher training. I have learned more about myself in the past seven months than I ever have in my twenty-six years of life. I have learned that yoga is *so* much more than those awesome poses I saw online. It's more than getting on your mat and doing a handstand (although those are my favorite). I've learned that yoga is love. Yoga is gratitude. Yoga is acceptance. Yoga for me now is taking a step back in a stressful situation and taking a huge breath. It is holding space for those who just need to get it off their chest. Yoga is being grateful for the smallest of things, like the smell of rain when it's much needed, abandoned kittens that become the love of your life, and the life-lasting friendships that mean so much. Yoga is life, and it is the most beautiful thing.

The Future

I see yoga in my future every day. I see the steps I'm taking and the things I do now, carrying my yoga practice very far into my future. I see myself pouring out any little bit of yoga knowledge I can to anyone who cares to listen. I can see myself investing in organizations and people who don't have yoga as accessible to them as some people do. I can even see myself teaching yoga in the most random places.

Yoga has helped me grow so much that I want to be able to give it to any and everyone who wants and needs this practice in their lives. Whether I teach them a breathing technique or a few simple postures to help them release some tension, I want to be able to do that. Giving what I have learned to others from this experience is where I see yoga playing the biggest role in my future.

The World

I want to see yoga E V E R Y W H E R E! I want to see it offered in schools, nursing homes, parks in the middle of the busiest cities, and in offices after work hours. I just want it everywhere because I believe it is needed everywhere. If it's space being held for someone in the middle of a library or a young student being shown how to do downward facing dog during gym class, I want to see that. I want to see someone take a deep, cleansing breath before they walk into their first day of college in a new place and the comfort of yoga wash over them. I want to see a woman shed her trauma while in her very first savasana. Plain and simple, I want to see yoga in every little corner of this big, big world. And now that I have knowledge of yoga and will continue to learn all that I can about it, I will make it my mission to share even the smallest piece of yoga to everyone I encounter. Here's to spreading the love that is yoga, one smile at a time.

Notes of Gratitude

A huge piece of gratitude goes to my friend, Blossom, who introduced me to yoga. She took me to my first class and encouraged me along the way. If it wasn't for her, I never would be on this beautiful path.

I also extend my love and many, many thanks to every teacher who has taken the time and held space for me when I needed it the most. Through the toughest times of my life, they gave me what I needed most—yoga.

My gratitude for my Yoga Mat family is always getting larger and larger, as they have *always* been there for me and given me the little, loving nudges I've needed to believe in myself. I have the biggest space for them in my heart.

I pour out gratitude to my teacher, Kelsy, a person I've felt so connected to since the very first moment I met her. She is the biggest ray of sunshine I have ever met in my life and has reassured me that I am not alone. My love for her is like family, and I will always hold a special place in my heart for her, for she has taught me some of the most profound things in my life.

I send out all of my thanks and love to my two amazing parents. Without their love, understanding, and support, I wouldn't be where I am today. Thank you for letting me stumble and fall, and being the ever-present hands that were always there to help me up. I don't think that I could ever thank you both enough for loving me despite my flaws or going along with all of my crazy ideas. I love you guys so big!

And my very highest, beyond highest form of love and gratitude, goes to Will, the man, who from day one, never loosened his grip on my hand. He makes sure that I know he loves me every day. The man who picked me up when I was at rock bottom and carried me for a very long time, he is the reason I am here today. He is my number one fan, my biggest motivator, my absolute best friend. Thank you, thank you, thank you. I could never say that enough.

From Light to Dark
Nonfiction by Amanda Rush

This project of writing my yoga story was extremely difficult for me. I started and stopped writing numerous times. I had these grandiose ideas of what I wanted this story to be. In the end, it turned out to be what it needed to be. I realized that I have been carrying around this deep heaviness that was the result of my wounding. I've been carrying it around as if it were this badge of honor, not wanting to let go of it because it was who I was. I'm ready to let it go. It has served its purpose. My mom had cancer, and after she had it for eight years, my mom died. During those eight years and the two that followed, I lost all four grandparents, my mother, my father, and my godmother. That decade of loss left its mark. From the age of seventeen until twenty-seven, I knew only suffering and death. Everyone that I ever loved and cared about left me. They left me to figure out life on my own. I often wondered who I would be now if that had not happened. Where would I be? I've come to the conclusion after all of those years of wondering, I AM who I'm supposed to be and exactly where I'm supposed to be.

Yoga found me in the deepest, darkest hole of my existence. To look at me back then and to know me, you would have never known I was struggling. Nobody knew how far gone I was, not even the closest of friends. Not even my husband. On the outside, everything looked normal, but beneath the surface there was a heaviness. A deep wounding. I didn't know who I was. Why was I here? What good could I do in the world when I wasn't even living in the world anymore, but merely surviving? I spent almost a decade of my life trying to save the ones I cared about most.

While everyone else my age was experiencing college and discovering who they were, I was working two jobs, playing a college sport on scholarship, and watching my family fall apart. All of my efforts to keep things together seemed a waste, for I couldn't save any of them. I spent a good portion of the years that followed running from the nightmare that had been my life. I was lost, broken, afraid, disconnected, and hopeless. I never thought I would ever feel normal again. Whole again. I was so tired of running. So tired of avoiding.

Yoga found me in the coldest part of the winter and darkest part of the year when the sun has retreated to the other side of creation. It found me hiding from the life that I didn't want to live anymore. Sleeping. Sleeping. Always sleeping. I was hoping that the thoughts in my head would stay quiet. I was wondering if this would be the last winter that I would see, and somewhere, deep down, finding comfort in that possibility. I could quiet the thoughts in my head most of the year. I was keeping busy with sports and work, and walking for miles and miles and miles with music drowning everything out. Yet in those quiet, sleepy, cold months of winter, it was impossible. The darkness always came for me in the winter. It wrapped around me like a warm blanket and would rock me in its arms and whisper its lies to me.

"There is no hope for you," it would say. "You are worthless, with nothing to give. There is no light.

The invitation came by text message. "Let's go do hot yoga," it read. I had looked into doing yoga just a month before but was scared off by what I found on the internet. And, here it was coming around again. I decided to try it out. Maybe it could be something to help drown out my thoughts, I figured. Or help with the physical pain that I was in from all of the running away from things I had been doing over the last ten years. I had a semi-frozen shoulder, sciatica, bulging discs, and a torn knee.

And, there was the voice again, the darkness saying, "You can't do yoga when you can't even stand up straight. You are weak."

I went to the yoga class anyway. I got overheated and fell out in the first ten minutes. There, I lay, in a sweaty heap on my yoga mat, fading in and out of blackness, fighting back tears of anger, frustration, embarrassment, and failure. I found my breath. In and out, in and out. I fought the urge to vomit. More breath. In and out, in and out. I fought the urge to run out of the room. Breathing in and out. Slowly, I rose to my feet. With my vision clearing and heart rate back to normal, I continued my practice. Lying in my very first savasana at the end of class, completely melted to the floor, a fire ignited deep within me. My competitive nature reawakened. I wanted to try this again.

With this small flame of light flickering deep inside of me, I scheduled my next class hoping to fan the flame of determination within me to light my way out of the darkness, out of the abyss. The darkness would not be so easily swayed. In the coming days, the temperature dropped to all-time lows, and with it, snow. There was enough snow to blanket everything in a deep pristine white and enough snow to close the yoga studio. That was enough snow to dampen my light. I retreated back to the couch, under the warmth and security of my blanket and the darkness held me close. When the fits of crying would come or the feeling of being so overwhelmed with depression, I would close my eyes and breathe. In and out. In and out. Each breath fanned that small ember that had ignited in the yoga class. I made a deal with myself. Each day after work I would go to my safe place on the couch and sleep, but only if I got up in time to catch the last yoga class of the night. No matter the temperature outside or bad weather, I would bundle myself up and go.

Each night, I would don my yoga gear and look at myself in the mirror and the lies would creep into my thoughts, *You're too fat for yoga pants. You look awful in yoga clothes. They're all going to laugh at you.*

Shaking off the thoughts, I would put on my Superman jacket and as I zipped it up, the two halves of the "S" crest would meet right over my heart and become whole. Superman had always been a symbol of strength for me. As a kid, I would sit and watch the movies over and over. He was my hero. He stood for everything I wanted to be when I grew up. If goofy klutzy Clark Kent could turn into Superman, then anyone could. Superman stood for truth, justice, and the American way. He fought the forces of darkness to bring hope to the world, and he did it all unconditionally. My Superman jacket was my armor and my shield from the world. I didn't feel so broken in my jacket. I felt safe. So off I'd go night after night to hot yoga and vinyasa classes.

I continued to collapse during hot yoga from the heat and collapse in vinyasa from utter exhaustion. Still, I went back night after night. Those first few months were hard. I judged myself for not being skinny enough. I judged myself for falling out of poses when everyone else could hold them steady for what seemed like forever. I judged myself for not even being able to do one of the most basic poses, mountain pose. Feet together, rooted deeply on the mat. Legs engaged. Navel pulled in towards the spine. Shoulders roll up and back, pressing the shoulder blades together. Chest is open, and heart is shining. Extending fully from feet to crown of the head, as if a string was pulling you up towards the ceiling, you stand. Palms gently open facing forward. One solid line of energy runs from head to toe. Seems pretty simple, standing up straight and yet I couldn't do it.

We were told in our yoga classes that there was no expectation, no competition, and to practice *ahimsa*, meaning nonviolence to one's self and to others. We were free to explore our edge but to not push past it. I fought many battles on my yoga mat those first months. There was the battle of will and of ego. The battle of acceptance—accepting my body the way it was on any given day and being mindful of its limitations. I was fighting anger and self-loathing and the idea of not being enough. I was searching for meaning and purpose.

It is hard to let go. It's hard to just accept what is. It's so much easier to accept the illusion of what isn't. It's hard to hold up a mirror and look into it and dare yourself to see the beautiful soul you are rather than the broken torn up mess you think you are. Yoga—the union of body and mind—strips away all which is false, leaving only the light of truth.

The more I went to yoga, the more I wanted yoga. I found myself getting to class earlier and earlier so I would have more time to just lie on my mat before class and be in the room. Finding my breath, I was finding my prana, my life force energy. In those moments when I let everything go, and gave everything up to the breath, I found the presence of God in my yoga practice. I found the divine light that balanced out the darkness. As the months went by, I began feeling lighter and lighter. Each night, I was leaving just a little bit more on my yoga mat. I was laying my burdens down one by one.

In our studio, we have a banner on the wall. It says, "I will catch you if you fall" – Yoga Mat. My yoga mat has collected sweat, tears, pain, anger, frustration, and everything else that no longer serves my greater good.

As the months went by, I felt myself opening up in so many different ways. Released from its burdens, my body began to find strength, stability, and movement. The breath flowed freely throughout my body, bringing with it a fluidity of movement. I felt less pain and restriction and found myself able to go deeper into the poses that I could barely hold before.

Off the mat, in my daily life, I realized that I was living more freely, not feeling bound up and shielding my heart from others, but rather shining bright for all to see. I was finding patience and compassion for others where I used to lash out in anger and judgment. I was coming into the studio with head held high with a smile on my face instead of trudging through the door with my head down and avoiding contact with others. I realized during those months that I wasn't alone in my struggles. We were all coming to our mats to work on something and through something. I began staying after class to chat with others. I started signing up for workshops and events, becoming more integrated into this collective and feeling linked together on a deeper level.

The turning point for me came when I made the decision to cut my beach vacation three days short so that I could come back to go on a three-day yoga retreat. To leave my friends, whom I had known for a decade, at the beach for this group of people whom I hardly knew, I realized that something had shifted in me and that I was headed down a new path in my life. Somewhere in those eight months of yoga, I found my direction.

One night during our evening meal, we were asked to name our favorite yoga pose. As we went around the table, poses such as tree, pigeon, warrior 2, dancer, and bird of paradise were called out. When it was my turn, I paused for a moment and said, "Mountain pose." Everyone kind of chuckled because it was so ordinary. I explained my hatred for that pose in the beginning because I couldn't do it. Life had beaten me down to the point where I literally could not stand up anymore. I walked with my head down, my heart tucked deep into the back of my chest, shoulders hunched over, and bent over at the waist, completely collapsed. Somewhere, in those eight months of yoga, I found my foundation. I found my strength and I broke the chains of despair that had bound me so tightly. I could finally stand on my own two feet again, shoulders pulled back and down, chest open and heart shining with my head held high. I no longer stood in mountain pose, I *was* the mountain. Strong, stable, and grounded.

Not long after the retreat, the yoga studio offered a special type of class on a Friday night. It was different than any other class they had offered before. It was a ninety-minute class done in a circle and they incorporated Thai massage, aromatherapy, energy healing, and meditation. I took the class and went home. I felt different after leaving the studio and was wandering around the house trying to pinpoint what it was. I lay down on the couch. It was the same couch that I ran to so often to hide myself from the world. I lay there taking stock of the evening and in quiet contemplation as the breath flowed in and out, I realized what had changed. During that ninety-minute class, I found peace. Lying there on the couch, the blanket of darkness that so many times enveloped me had been replaced by the warm divine light of unconditional love and acceptance. The lies of illusion were no longer free-flowing through my mind. All that was there was truth in the stillness of my mind. I was whole, not broken. I was wounded deeply through life's experiences in order to allow my inner light to shine outward as a beacon of hope to others who have lost their way in the darkness.

As my one year yoga anniversary approached, a change in ownership at my studio threatened its existence. One evening after class in a moment that was a combination of joking and desperation, my yoga teacher and new studio owner asked if I'd like to buy into a yoga studio partnership. Without hesitation and without thought, I said, "Yes." That night, our partnership was formed. People often ask how I could make such a decision on a whim, without taking time to weigh any of the potential outcomes of that decision. My answer to that question was, and still is, that on some level I have been waiting my entire life for that question to be asked. This is my dharma, what I am meant to do with my life.

To say yoga changed my life is a massive understatement. Yoga transformed me into who I am today. It has become my life-defining moment. I had no idea how to run a business, but I accepted the challenge because I knew deep down on a soul level that I was meant to be there. Owning this business opened my eyes up to a whole new realm of possibilities. I wanted to learn so much more.

Yoga transformed my life, but how did it happen? People say, "Yoga does what yoga does." I wanted to know how and why. I was once asked to describe yoga in one word. The word I chose was "Magic."

All of my life, I yearned for a deeper understanding of spiritual connection. I always believed in something bigger than myself but could never quite fit what that was in a box because the box always seemed to be too small to contain the wonder that is the divine. These words so eloquently sung by Bono in the song by U2, "I believe in Kingdom Come, then all the colors will bleed into one. But yes, I'm still running. You broke the bonds and loosed the chains. Carried the cross of my shame, you know I believe it. But I still haven't found what I'm looking for. But I still haven't found what I'm looking for..." were my anthem for most of my life. I was searching for meaning and purpose in this life and not finding it. Yoga opened that door for me and when I walked through it, it changed my life.

I always believed in the idea of extreme possibilities but never imagined that the idea could turn into my reality. Almost immediately after signing the ownership papers, a new level of awareness opened itself up to me. It was as if by signing that contract, I was agreeing to take responsibility and guardianship over some of life's most wondrous and fantastical elements of the metaphysical world. I was introduced to reiki and energy medicine, healing through sound vibration, and the healing and protective properties of crystals and other stones. Our studio not only became a place to come and do yoga, but it became a healing space with healing for everyone on all levels.

As yoga students, we are taught to set an intention for our practice at the beginning of each class. The word "intention" did not become fully realized in my mind until I saw the proof of what setting an intention could achieve. We set the intention for our business to be that place where people can go to heal. For those who seek it, to have a safe and loving environment to lay down their armor and find peace and healing by reconnecting the body and mind through breath. People started coming through our doors to find that healing, and others came through our doors to facilitate the healing.

Synchronicity is defined as the simultaneous occurrence of events that appear significantly related but have no discernible causal connection. I always wanted to believe that everything was connected, but I didn't truly believe that it was possible until it became a daily routine. Anytime there has been a need, that need has been met by someone or something. By filling our studio space with unconditional love and acceptance to all, we are manifesting the change we want to see in the world. All of those spiritual aspects that I knew were there but couldn't reach were revealed to me only when I was ready. And when I was ready, the door blew wide open.

After only experiencing yoga for ten months, I became a yoga studio owner. After owning a yoga studio for a year, I started my teacher training to be a yoga teacher. My expectations were so high going into teacher training. I wanted to know everything. I wanted to be introduced to all aspects of yoga. There had been opportunities during my journey to do a teacher training but something held me back from going down that path at the time. I know now it was because I wasn't ready then. Those teacher trainings would not have resonated with me. By waiting, I was able to take the training when I was truly open and ready to live the experience.

We were told that something somewhere within the training would resonate with us. It would speak to us on a deep level and only then would we know where our passion for this work would pull us. Apart from our teacher training, a kundalini instructor that studied under Yogi Bajan came to us for a few months and taught at the studio, and I fell in love with kundalini yoga. She introduced us to gong meditation and mantra meditation as well, and all of that deeply resonated with me. Her visit was followed by teacher training weekends that introduced holistic medicine, Qi-gong, meridians, and chakras, and I just couldn't get enough. Now, I want to learn about shamanic healing and Native American healing. I want to study Qi-Gong. I want to study kundalini yoga. I want to learn more about holism and mysticism. I want to be a healer.

As my three-year yoga anniversary is approached, I looked back on my journey and was amazed at the transformation. I still wear my Superman jacket and my Superman t-shirts. That "S" on my chest that shielded me from the world, now shines so brightly, illuminated by the divine light that pours from my heart. The scars of my wounding are ripped open for that light to shine. I am bringing hope to those that have lost their light.

My mother instilled upon us the love of music. She would sing to us, and she taught us to play her favorites songs on the guitar. Somewhere along the way, I lost that. The memory of those moments was too painful, I suppose. I caught myself not too long ago, humming to myself a familiar song that I must have heard a million times when I was younger. "This little light of mine, I'm going to let it shine. Let it shine, let it shine, let it shine." I stand here today with gratitude for the darkness. Gratitude for the wounding and the loss I have endured. I walk my path fully embraced by the light and when darkness comes into my path, I will take what it gives me and use it as an offering to bring more light into the world and to hold the space for others. I will provide a healing place for others to see and recognize the goodness and light within themselves. That is my dharma.

"And just as the Phoenix rose from the ashes, she too will rise. Returning from the flames, clothed in nothing but her strength more beautiful than ever before."—Unknown

Breathe Deeply
Poetry by Brittany Howard

The feeling of deep sadness is not all-consuming.
It is not a constant umbrella of tears; it is a deep,
deep heaviness within the body that when you pause,
you feel its weight
bearing down on the space between the chest and abdomen,
in the space where the top ribs part directions away from each other.
It is a tightening you suffer that brings the shoulder blades
around the body,
as if trying to hug the solar plexus in sympathy.

The collarbones melt down the chest, relentlessly weighing down
upon the torso. The heaviness sinks and sinks within the body
until it travels all the way through to the flexed spine,
throbbing in agony, hunched over to endure the weight
of repressed sorrow.
The core of the body aches in distress
for the burden of a deeply wounded soul.

Somewhere, slipping between the collapsed muscles and bones,
the breath begins to flow and fill,
gliding down the esophagus, pooling beneath the chin.
With a powerful inhale, the chest and head begin to rise,
the shoulder blades slide back into place
while the solar plexus starts to ascend.
Agonizing pain uproots from the spine, allowing the back body
to shift naturally; the deep sadness floats to the surface of the skin,
riding a wave of breath lightly upon the space surrounding the heart.

Each inhale floats up,
each exhale sinks down,
and each breath keeps the pain from sinking back into the body below.

Scars Full of Light
Nonfiction by Jessica Gibbs

Journal Entry 4/23/16
Some scars you see from the outside and you know the person has been through a lot of pain and, likely, suffering. Other scars lie hidden internally. It's harder to see those journeys, sometimes even for the person on the journey. You don't notice these scars, or you push it down until it is so far gone, you can almost forget about it.

11 years earlier
I waited for the blow to come to my face. He hadn't hit me before, but he also had never shoved me into a wall and yanked my hair. I felt his fingers tighten around my chin and cheek as his soft, brown eyes turned nearly black. I could feel his breath across my face, minty and cool, despite the moment.

Then, my eyes flew open, my breath became shallow, and my heart pounded in my chest. The whirling air of the fan made the tears sting across my cheeks. I realized it was only a dream. Only a dream. A dream that had once been a reality. A real part of life I had buried deep inside.

Almost out of habit, I turned over to look at my forearms, half expecting to see fading, yellow finger imprints. The ones I would have to cover with long sleeves. And even to this day, I usually wear long sleeves, even in the throes of summer when it is over ninety degrees outside.

I sat up in bed, leaning my back to the wall and hugging my knees to my chest. I remembered how he'd made me throw all my clothes away. All the tops and skirts that were too revealing or "slutty." He would replace them with designer sweaters and jeans, flowers and trips. Really a dream come true at the time, if it had not ended up being such a nightmare.

He somehow chipped away at my sense of self. I went from free-spirited and sassy, with a laugh that would fill a whole room, to a meek shell of a person who was constantly begging for forgiveness. Forgiveness for being partnered with a male colleague in class. Forgiveness for missing a phone call. Forgiveness for going out to a club and wearing his favorite dress. Over time, my self-love and confidence faded, being replaced by this new twisted sense of love. Endless gestures, gifts, and texting. Constant reassurances of love. And broken thoughts of myself. I never seemed to be enough. I was constantly trying to get back into his good graces in order to have a good day as a couple.

Then, the relationship abruptly ended. He ended it after cheating on me, and I still begged him to take me back. Before this relationship, I could never understand why abused women would stay with their abusers, but now I get it. It's a slow process of brain washing, one that gradually takes you down to your lowest point, but you don't even realize because you are still admiring all the glitter from above. Once you hit rock bottom, you're desperately trying to hold on because you know no other way out.

Even after we had broken up, he continued to call me, whispering how he missed me and how he still dreamt of a life together. How much he still loved me. I held onto the hope that he did still love me because I did not have any love for myself. This back and forth act went on for a few weeks, until one fateful evening he asked for advice about his newfound relationship. A relationship coincidentally with the girl he had slept with while we were together.

I snapped back to my sassy self in that moment.

"I don't ever want to talk to you again. I'm done. This is over," I said, slamming the phone down.

He called over twenty times and left half a dozen voicemails that night, pleading and confessing his love. I never responded and felt waves of anger and hurt wash over me with each call.

A few weeks later, the voicemails continued but his tactic had changed.

"Jess, I love you. You know that. If you don't take my calls, I will come down there. I will find you, and I will make you listen," he said in a cool tone, the one I knew meant trouble.

Those voicemails sent chills down my spine and caused me to panic. I began looking over my shoulder at school and the grocery store. I looked under my car when leaving my house. I ended up moving and changing my number. The prickly feeling of someone stalking me lasted for more than six months but faded gradually with time, and life moved on. I never let on to friends or family the terror I felt, and I made myself busy with finishing graduate school. I did not have time to process those emotions *and* earn a graduate degree.

Although the relationship was over, the scars that came with it followed me. I let them fester for over a decade. Any time a thought or feeling would come from that dark, hurt place, I would be too busy to notice. I needed to be too busy to notice, lest I go to the deep place of self-hatred.

After this relationship, I desperately sought love and attention from each new romantic relationship I entered. I ignored my intuition whispering in my ear that this person or that person was not for me and proceeded without caution, valuing love of another over love for myself. I fractured myself with each relationship, becoming whatever I thought might entice a potential mate. And, it worked temporarily. I had a fairytale wedding and began working toward the goal of settling into a life with a house, a dog, and 2.5 kids. I ignored the thoughts that this life was not the life I dreamed of and focused on thoughts of finding happiness in the status quo.

I had happy moments in my marriage, but it was not meant to last. Three years into it, my husband decided to move to the Midwest for a job opportunity. Every fiber in my body screamed, "No," yet I went anyway, determined to save the marriage and succeed at being a wife. I was terrified that if this marriage failed, I would not find love again.

After moving, I signed up for yoga classes online to pass the time because I had no job. I had gone from being successful to unemployed. My already fragile self-confidence plummeted. My family doubted me for moving with my husband. I felt such guilt. Guilty because I did not want to move. Guilty because I was letting myself down. Guilty because I wasn't being supportive of my husband.

With the newfound online yoga classes, I pounded out vinyasas on the mat, taking as many classes as I could handle until falling asleep in corpse pose. Conversations between me and my husband became stilted. Laughter faded between us. I would come to my mat and face-plant while attempting one-legged flying crow, which I had no business doing as a beginner, but I also had no idea that I should not be attempting this pose. As I would come crashing down, time and time again, I'd collapse into fits of laughter on the mat. Yoga had brought me joy again and made me feel lighter each time I placed my feet on the cushy green cells of the mat.

When I started my practice, all I knew about yoga was that there were poses and everyone seemed to speak about gratitude. I knew little of myself and certainly did not feel grateful for where life had taken me. My sense of self had gotten lost somewhere between the abuse and a "safe" marriage to a kind husband who wasn't actually my kind at all. Yet, I did not open *that* box. Better to keep it tucked away and keep a smile on my face while I looked for jobs and tried to learn Sanskrit.

I finally found several contract jobs in my field. Once I started working, I began practicing various yoga poses on my breaks, feeling a rush of exhilaration to do yoga in public with the risk of getting caught. Yoga had become my entertainment, my exercise, and my life. My husband couldn't understand why I always wanted to practice. He couldn't understand this new online community of friends I had found through social media. With the silence of my marriage growing deafening each day, I needed those friends and their kind words. I would spend endless hours typing back responses of support as my husband watched TV. The social media outlet also allowed me to avoid facing myself. It was a virtual place where I could be happy.

After a harsh Midwest winter, my practice shifted toward heart openers. I read about chakras and how the heart chakra's color is green. With the increase in heart openers, I began to notice green everywhere that spring—from the buds on trees to flowers poking their way through the grass. I felt a shift happening within that I associated with my heart slowly starting to open, like one of the tightest buds on the tree outside the apartment window.

Coinciding with all the green and heart chakra work, my backbend practice also began to change. The tightness around my shoulders decreased. I found my breath when my hands touched my feet in kapotasana, a pose that had made my head hurt and left me breathless just months before.

All of these changes brought about a sense of peace and awareness I had never before encountered. I not only wanted to know more about yoga, but needed something more than just the physical. I wanted to know more about myself, and with each heart opener, I noticed there were dark scars within me. I felt a transformation occurring. A transformation I did not understand and one that would not be satisfied by a solely physical practice. I impulsively bought a mala one evening and delved into reading about meditation and healing. I started using the mala and mantras, flicking the beads one by one between my middle finger and thumb, feeling slightly ashamed that I couldn't sit on the floor to meditate, but rather I sat on a stool.

Shortly after buying the mala, I purchased an app for meditation and did it nightly, sitting on the toilet with the lid down. Alone in the bathroom, I could detach from my thoughts of worthlessness and hatred for myself. Alone in the bathroom, I didn't have to face my failing marriage and all the disappointments of my life. Yet, through meditation, I was gradually beginning to face myself and shine a light on my scars.

My husband and I began going to marriage counseling shortly after I began meditating. I could see that I was lost. I could also see that I had been playing the victim card to myself, blaming the past for my unhappiness in the present. Over the course of the counseling sessions, my counselor gave me additional positive mantras to try. I wrote them ten times each, filling one whole spiral bound page daily. I also wrote positive qualities about myself on my mirror and read them aloud to myself each morning upon her suggestion. Initially, I could not meet my eyes in the mirror, tears welling up as I tried to say the words, "I am kind" and continue down the list of qualities. When I could not meet my own eyes in the mirror, the truth hit me, causing my chest to tighten. I not only did not like what I saw, but I had a sense of hatred toward myself. It was not the words from the abusive relationship that were hurting me. It was me, going to war and attacking every bit of myself each day. With that realization, I slid to the tiled bathroom floor, shuddering sobs and wracking my body for the next ten minutes until I had to leave for work.

After that tearful morning, I was determined to return to loving and appreciating myself. I began going to counseling alone, working through the past issues of emotional abuse I had not realized were affecting me. I continued my physical practice and renewed my vow to meditate each day. Meditating daily allowed me to distance myself from the scars of the past. I became able to observe those dark places from a distance. I also continued the positive mantras and worked on taking slow, deep breaths while walking down this unknown road toward myself, scars and all. As I stumbled along this road, I sifted through pieces of the old me, the woman who had become someone else, and found gems of the real me on the wayside. These gems were the ones I held onto, knowing they were my soul.

My sense of self and self-confidence increased with my yoga practice. I grew bolder and attempted a drop back into upward facing bow. I also grew braver off the mat and asked for a divorce. The act of starting over was terrifying, but once the decision was made, an enormous weight was lifted, and my chest began to expand fully with each breath. With meditation, I grew daring enough to shine a light into the crevices within that held the scars of the past.

Once the decision to divorce was final, I left the Midwestern apartment and town where my life fell apart. I sold nearly everything I owned, hanging onto a few pieces of furniture, my yoga mat and mala in order to create a new life. I felt grateful for finding a road leading toward myself via a green yoga mat rolled out amidst the rubble of a failed marriage and crushed dreams.

I practiced daily once my marriage was over, weaving poses into all the hardships. The day I left my previous life, I felt the bumpity bump bump of a flat tire not even a mile from my old apartment. I chose to do an upward facing bow on that flat tire, my brother-in-law watching me in amusement. I wanted to sit down and cry with frustration because I could not seem to get a mile away from my past before failing, but somehow, a heart opener is what came to me in that moment instead of tears.

As I drove across the country to a new, unknown life, handstands were had in the grass with my niece and nephew in West Virginia. A day later, an eagle pose felt right at a gas station while filling up the tank.

And another handstand with the repairman for my cracked windshield, which coincidentally happened the day I arrived at my new apartment. Yoga had taught me strength and perseverance no matter what the day may bring. It had taught me to trace my way back to my breath and observe the lesson in the moment.

Not all the moments were happy or silly. I cried in pigeon pose countless times in my new apartment, surrounded by a few empty boxes and a mattress on the floor. I lay breathless on the mat after moving into dwi pada dandasana, feeling the exhilaration of my heart opening to new possibilities. And, if I'm honest, I fell asleep more times than I'd care to admit in savasana.

Yoga became central to my life. I practiced yoga at lunch. At work. At home. In public. Everywhere. I meditated daily. Sometimes even twice when the day was full of extra stress. Yoga was magical. I had somehow transformed my greatest sorrow into my greatest happiness. I had turned hate into love. I found gratitude in my work—a job I had previously moaned about now brought tears of joy to my eyes each week.

It was not only I who noticed the changes. People around me pointed out how I seemed "calmer" and more "grounded." Families of patients I treated would say, "You really enjoy your job. I can tell." They were right. This practice of yoga—the breath, the poses, the meditation—had transformed me. I became less anxious, more self-loving and overall, more able to give. And most importantly, I had found my sense of Self again.

I took almost a year to heal after the divorce, taking my daily vitamin dosage of yoga, meditating, and spending vast stretches of time alone, journaling, and writing. As I dived into learning all I could about yoga and healing, I began to consider a teacher training to deepen my practice. I started meditating with mantras of Kuan Yin and wore my mala everywhere.

Meditation led me to explore and appreciate the shadows of myself and others. I became less afraid of the dark scars and memories from the past and came to appreciate each of them, realizing my strength had come from some of the darkest scars. Each of these scars carried a lesson. Each lesson was necessary for my growth. With this shift in thinking, my scars became full of light. Each dark crevice became a place of uncharted territory to learn more about myself.

With all of these lessons and changes, I continued wanting to learn more, wanting to go further down this road of exploration of myself. In 2016, I decided to move forward with a Yoga Teacher Training (YTT). I sold my wedding band and engagement ring to cover the cost with my ex-husband's blessing. I worked my 9 to 5 (actually 8 a.m.-6:30 p.m. or later) and practiced until midnight during the week and attended YTT each Friday through Sunday. I began believing in the power of intention and speaking goals into action. I noticed my negative thoughts related to myself were becoming less. Yoga had given me confidence, gratitude, and the ability to sit with myself. I no longer spent energy hating my body or myself. I continued to work on not feeling impatient with myself and trusting that I was exactly where I needed to be. I no longer played the victim card, and instead felt empowered by all the events in my life.

I've returned to my sassy, playful self, and I love her fiercely. My laughter fills the room again, bouncing off the walls. I've found comfort in the breath and often take time to slow my breathing when I feel tension creeping into my shoulders. The anxious tone in my journal has softened into feelings of gratitude and love.

Journal entry Jan 9, 2017 (after yoga teacher training)
"Cause it's you, it's you that you're running from," *Signs of Light* by The Head and the Heart.
Monday Feels. I've heard this song dozens of times, but today it took me back in time.
I used to run from myself. Distracted by degrees, social circles, awards, physical endeavors, and so on. Until life turned me upside down. Broke me. I couldn't run anymore. The only option I had was to go within and figure out why life wasn't working. I looked every day at myself (literally and within). I read books. Went to counseling. Meditated. Anything and everything to heal, I did. And one day, the tears stopped. I ripped away every bit of the old life that wasn't me and started over.

I've never wanted to go back, but I am grateful for it all. The lessons. The healing. The love. And finding myself again...

Thank you, Yoga, for saving me and guiding me back to my Self. Thank you for showing me that my scars are full of light.

Settled
Poetry by Yvette Huber

Knees and hips,
Worn and creaky.
Back and shoulders,
Stiff and battered.
My ego settles for yoga.

But my head is stuck
In a gymnastics routine.
Doubts flip and tumble.
Feet struggle to stick
The landing of each pose.

I settle for holding back.
Tuck my pride
Into Child's Pose,
And my heart
Rattles the rib cage.

Anticipating
Round Two,
I unfold my body to
Smooth out a wrinkle
Of self-judgment.

Still impatient
To win the battle,
I wrestle my limbs into a bind.
I hold too tightly to letting go.
Stalemate.

I settle for modification.
Unencumbered,
My body unwinds its tension.
Punishing thoughts unravel,
And my heart unlocks.

Open to possibility
In this practice.
Buoyed by my breath.
Steady and at ease.
I am settled.

Love, Connection, Healing, and Magic
Nonfiction by Erika Wolfe

Yoga. Prana. Asana. Vinyasa. Chakras. Energy. Yamas. Peace. Love.

I could go on and on with these words that were a foreign language. I had no clue what any of it was or even meant until the invitation to attend a hot yoga class. That's all it took to jump start me into living my life's purpose and mission which is to nurture and encourage the journey to one's true self. My dharma.

All I knew up until then was a shit storm. Not really a pleasant thing to visualize, I mean, *who really throws shit into a storm or even wants to stand in all that?* I was a mess. Life was a mess, and I had no idea how far I had fallen and how broken I was. In hindsight, I know that I had to travel through that crazy storm in order to stand in the space where I am now, and own it. I am who I am because of my shit storm. Thank you. I give gratitude and humbly acknowledge that it was all for a reason.

My growing up years were filled with a lot of alone time, and not much love. My family never said, "I love you." We never hugged or showed affection, some of the things I desperately wanted and needed. I grew up knowing I wasn't "good enough," and I am not sure if I ever did anything to gain the approval I craved. Goodness, looking back, my family missed out on a lot of love. They didn't know what they hadn't learned. Later, my yoga practice taught me how to forgive.

Marriage to a soldier followed and the kids shortly thereafter. All I ever wanted was to be a good wife and mom. I loved every moment. Then, war happened. That was the beginning of the end of what I now call my former life. A decade followed, filled with way too much trauma for all four of us.

Our little unit was torn apart by a wound so hidden and invisible that it was a secret buried deep within my husband. No doctor, no medicine, nothing explained the shit storm that grew and grew. The words I clung to were, "This is not the man I fell in love with. Something is wrong." The puzzle was missing a piece. Abuse became a part of that puzzle. Not just one or two, but too many kinds. I watched as our kids began to hate him. I hated him. We all became so disconnected. My son turned to drugs. My daughter turned to alcohol and self-harming. I turned to working myself to death, existing, and not living. We were a hot mess. A well kept secret—on the outside we looked like the somewhat perfect family. It's amazing how we can fool ourselves.

A series of events caused the storm to throw out lightning bolts, and post-traumatic stress disorder (PTSD) and traumatic brain injury (TBI) became household names and more acronyms for us. Finally, the missing piece was found. My husband spilled his secret and by sharing, we lost him. The secret kept him in the present moment, fighting it every day. Once he let go, his mind took him to his safe space, a time in his life before he was ever hurt, to an eight year old. It took some time to put the next puzzle together to understand why and how this all happened.

I called the kids home, while their Dad was fighting the war in his reality. He surrounded himself with his safety measures, guns, and hunting knives. *Seriously, what the hell was happening?* It was a matter of a few days, not weeks, that so much happened. I had to connect to the kids—I couldn't do this alone. They learned about the missing puzzle piece. By the time this blew up, they had almost disowned him, but they rallied together and showed up to support and love their Dad. I was so proud of my kids. I became a caregiver, no longer a wife. The kids even stepped into parenting roles for their Dad.

In addition, I realized I had lost me. *When did I lose me...?* The loving, joyful, happy, giving human was no longer inside me. I had become sad, lost, and broken—a shell. I was in a new shit storm. I had nothing else to lose. I had thought back then that I lost it all already. My husband was gone. Not in the physical sense, but he was gone mentally. The Army, war, PTSD, TBI, and a decade of hiding a secret had ravaged his body, mind, and soul. I had mourned the loss of him. My family was in shards. My children were a mess. We were all bleeding, metaphorically, and I couldn't hold anything together anymore. My friends slowly disappeared because I became that soul-sucking energy vampire. I was in too much sadness, devastated by what my life had become. I couldn't find a way out. Circling the drain of despair, there was no outlet to release the pressure. All of the things I once loved doing—gardening, building, dreaming, DIY-ing, yard saleing—were gone. A switch was flipped and my former life was done.

This is when my yoga journey started, on a September evening nearly four months after all of the aforementioned, and that was only in 2012. I did not have a clue what yoga was...it wasn't something I had ever done before nor had I looked into it to have any base knowledge. I had spent years in gyms, doing gym rat things, walking, weights, and machines. Yoga was not my thing, but I thought, *what the heck. Let's try.*

Then, yoga did what it does. I entered the yoga studio—a huge warehouse with a high ceiling. It was dark since there were no windows. *What do I do?* I was so nervous then, that I don't even remember if I had my own yoga mat or if I had to borrow one. I unrolled some mat next to Tammy's mat. She's my sister from another lifetime. She knew me better than anybody, and she was the one friend who held me up in my shit storm. Her daughters were there in the yoga warehouse. Their familiar faces brought comfort. Wy was there. She was this beautiful tattooed creature, who had invited the gang. She's the reason why I was there to begin with. Her invite was the one that unrolled into my life. (A beautiful story that travels into the future is for another day.)

I had no clue what I was doing that practice, but I fell in love, finding my outlet, and it was a slow and intense process. Before I knew it, yoga became my drug of choice. Yoga became my cure. My body, my higher self, was learning the ethics of yoga on its own, without ever reading a single yoga book. The yamas and niyamas were unfolding as was I, and I began to find kindness in myself. Compassion. Non-harming. Letting go. Finding moments of joy, exhaustion, and peace.

My journey left everything behind as a new chapter was written. I was changing and evolving. I wasn't understood by many. There were teachers that popped into my journey with the help, guidance, support, and love. More than once, I had been told by old friends that I was the glue that kept "us" all together, and now, *where was their glue?* They missed me, yet I couldn't go back. It was hard, seeing friendships that were thought to be for a lifetime fall apart.

Yoga was my friend now. Six to seven days a week my mat was unrolled for me to leave a little bit more of my *ick* on it. I was driven by a force within. My soul was screaming to be released from the hell it was in. Yoga was my glue. I couldn't be the glue for anybody. I had to learn how to glue myself back together. Little by little, with sweat, tears, and aches. My intention for months was "letting go," and yet, I had no clue what needed to be let go, though there was plenty. I was working hard on me.

In the meantime, and I didn't know this until much later, my dependence on my daughter's strength had sucked her dry. She was my rock for so long. Even though I was getting better, the damage had been done. The tree had been leaning on the sapling far too long and the sapling bent to the ground. It's her story to tell, and I am grateful that her guardian angels pulled her out. It wasn't her time to go.

I had introduced yoga to her, my daughter, a few months prior. I saw her grow. I saw her strength and beauty. I was in awe. I will never forget the practice when we both got into birds of paradise at the same moment and our teacher saw us. It was magic. She stepped away from everything—yoga and me, too, when she was broken. It was the worst time of my life. I lost her, and she disconnected from me. My heart was broken. She is everything to me. It was nearly a year before she allowed me back into her circle. It was the test of a lifetime. She did come back to yoga very slowly after that year.

In that time, all I had was my mat and the fever within to learn. *What was the magic behind all this?* I didn't understand. I was a sponge, thirsty for every drop of knowledge my yoga teachers shared in class. All I knew is what I learned on my mat. No book. No magazine. I didn't go searching for answers. The answer found me. A teacher training program opened up at my studio just five months into my yoga story. *What was I thinking? Could I?*

I don't think I intended to be a teacher, but I wanted to learn. From whom better than the ones who had helped me to grow? I was gluing myself together. By healing myself, I showed my daughter that I was capable of changing.

In my process, my therapist asked me, "Who are you?"

I didn't know. These words spilled out of my heart long ago:

Who am I?
Mom, wife, friend,
What dreams do I have?

To be happy, serene, loved, at peace.
I wish I didn't hurt my family with words when I feel unloved,
unwanted, or hurt.
I want to laugh and be happy again. I don't handle stress well. I used to
eat for stress now I don't care to eat at all.
I don't like my life.
I don't like being alone.
The hurt that I had felt is now replaced by a void that I have to figure
out how to fill.
The void has to be filled by things that make me happy and whole,
things that I want to do, be, and have.
My husband can't help me, neither can my daughter.
Maybe Frank's words, "follow your heart" will guide me to fill the void.
The hard part is waiting to see where this road will take me. I don't like
the unknown and emptiness I feel right now.
I will wait.
Sad, lonely, afraid, but I will wait because the day will come soon.
I hope that my heart will know where to go.

11 Mar 13

I introduced yoga to all those that would listen. Some came to try out a
class, some listened to me gush and gush. It was an obsession. I had to
be driving them nuts. I am guessing they were just happy I was in a
better place. Before I even read any required reading from my teacher
training, I was already going through the motions of forgiving myself.
My family. I was letting go. First it was emotions. Then the
attachments started. The biggest yard sale of my life unfolded. I wasn't
a hoarder by any means. I was a collector of many pretties. My monkey
mind had plans galore back in the day. Exhausting just thinking about
how I used to be. Exhausting how much stuff I had been holding onto,
in all aspects. I was so, so happy to be letting go.

Just a few months later, these words spilled from my soul:

Things that I love,
My husband, _____
My children, ____ and _____
My soon to be daughter-in-law

_____
My pets, all of them
My friends

And all the others I missed
My angel, Frank
I loved growing up in Germany.
I love pink, bright and vibrant.
I love the outdoors.
I love being outside, just being me.
New tattoos
I love learning all about yoga.
I love helping others.
I love when my husband knows what's wrong with me and tries to fix it.
I love that my daughter always helped me with my clothing styles. I am so plain. She makes me shine.
I love my son's goofiness and silliness that makes me smile.
YOGA!!
I love talking and being with my kids.
Canoeing!!
Scuba!!
Yard sales
Four leaf clovers for they make me think of my daughter.
Christmas vacation to PR, having the crazy family all together.
Having Vey as family therapist lol
I love books, all kinds.
I love the color of spring, flowers and leaves awakening.
I love being in touch with the "Universe."
I love the talks that I have with Tammy.
I love that I share the light thing with Tammy's parents.
The tattoos I share with my family, they all have a story.
YOGA!!
Love phone calls, not text messages.
I love that I am no longer sad.
I love that I can laugh and be happy.
I love that I am still a spitfire but a careful one.
Finally being able to love myself, which took awhile....
I love myself, I am me.
A new ME
Erika

June 13, 2013

JOY! Happy! Can you feel the energy shift? I would not have had a clue back then what an energy shift was. Growth.

Then, the breakup happened. My yoga studio and my teacher got "divorced." It was awful. My teacher training fell into a hole. My loyalty was being tested. *Where do I go? Who do I believe?* I saw what happened, and it broke my yoga heart in two. I walked away from my mat. I could not understand how the teachings of yoga that I strongly believed in were not observed. Devastated, I lost yet another relationship.

Months later, my studio owner reached out. She had seen my story unfold but didn't know the internal struggle I was dealing with. Her love brought me back. Little by little, I began to trust and believe there was hope. Soon thereafter, a new teacher training opportunity opened up. Without hesitation, I signed up. I wasn't done learning and growing. I struggled at the end of the training, and fear had a good hold on me. My heart was in it, but my mind was telling me that I wasn't good enough. My teachers knew and were sneaky in pushing me out into the limelight for me to shine. They saw what I did not see. I had become a yoga teacher that day, and I have loved every moment. I was what I wanted to be when I grow up. Finally, I figured it out. I learned to hold the space for transformation to happen, first for myself, then my practitioners. Recently these words, "when you find your cure, you want to share it with everybody," were shared with me. I certainly shared the love and cure.

Many new doors opened in this time of growth. I began my journey of becoming a practitioner of energy work in several modalities. Learning about the metaphysical world at a fast pace, the healing arts became another part of my story. There are so many trainings and not enough time. I couldn't read, learn, ingest, and share fast enough.

As life has it, the story was going to shift again, just when I thought it all was settled. My studio owner was ready to rest. Her story needed a break. She asked me...*would I consider holding the space for a yoga studio?* I don't think I even blinked an eye and said, "Yes." I knew what a healing place this studio was, and how important it was to continue holding the space for healing and transformation to happen.

My dharma unrolled that fall. I did not have a clue what owning and running a business meant. I only had a knowing in my heart that I was in the right place and everything was happening for a reason. Trusting and believing that it was all meant to be, it was. There were struggles along the way and lessons learned the hard way. The best decision that has ever happened to me, I knew with my heart and soul what this little studio was meant to be.

I began the business with two others, and sadly it didn't work out. As that story was very quickly ending, I jokingly and with some desperation asked my yogi student one evening, "Do you want to be an owner of a yoga studio?"

Without hesitation, she said, "Yes."

I had been her teacher for almost a year at that time, but we didn't "know" each other. There was never time in our stories to ever connect deeply. This was huge. Later that night, I messaged her saying, "You don't have to do this." However, she didn't back out. Her own healing story with yoga was enough to believe in our studio, and she believed in me.

My story is filled with a million moments of love from thereon. We filled our studio and community with love and hugs. Slowly, we manifested the space where like-minded people came together. We see the healing happen here every day. May it be in a smile, a bear hug, tears, or a yoga mat unrolled while its yogi is lying exhausted in savasana. The bright, shiny, smiley faces that come up from that pose are priceless.

I trust that everything happens for a reason and with unconditional love everything is possible. Believe. That is the magic of yoga, finding peace within.

You're not alone out there. I am right here. I will hold this space for you. My story isn't the same, but we have traveled a similar road, and have come out on the other side to be there for each other. It takes that one moment to change your life.

One yoga class is all it took, and my magic was unrolling itself with my mat. My healing began.

Metamorphosis
Poetry by Sheryl Hayes

As I lie chest deep in the earth
My mind rushes back to someone I know—
A vague vision of who "I" once was—
So many deep breaths ago.
Renewed and awakened through each exhale,
Limbs stretching past their normal boundary
To show this person now lying here—
She has surpassed the girl in her memory.
~~~
Every mold and fold, guided by an energy—
A force more powerful than her being,
Reminding her that her birth in womb and in practice
Has much life, purpose, and meaning.
Her flaws have become unrecognizable.
Negative talk has become just a whisper.
She is not worried about yesterday or tomorrow,
She has made peace with the Ego inside her.

Every Child Is Our Own
Nonfiction by E.W. Dziadon III

If you were raising your child in a war zone, how far would you go to ensure her health and safety? The average American will never know the fear and frustration of raising a child in a war zone. For the parents in war-torn Afghanistan, it is a daily norm. The amazing amount of courage, trust, and humility it takes to accept help for the sake of your child, your precious cargo to carry safely through this world, is something we all have in us.

When you're given a mission in the Army, you never know what may come your way. Why would this day be the exception? It was a normal July day in Bagram, Afghanistan, and the 120-day winds were lightly blowing their usual fifteen mile per hour, dust-laden way across the airfield. I, having charge of a CH-47 Chinook helicopter, had gone through the routine of preparing it for flight, conducting a crew brief, loading the day's cargo for delivery, and giving the standard safety brief to the passengers. Going through my superstitiously ritualistic last hugs of my soldiers that would be flying other helicopters, I felt confident that all the blocks were checked and we could embark on another scenic tour through the Afghan countryside. Once in the air, the guns were test fired, cargo was double checked for security, and a walk around the inside of the helicopter indicated that all was good to go.

Flying along low and fast at one hundred feet, to avoid exposure to long range weapons, the farmland of the Bagram valley passed underneath, giving one the unique experience of seeing the men toiling in their fields and women going about their daily duties within the protective fort-like walls of the family compound. The farmland gave way to sparsely wooded hillsides and eventually to the majestic Hindu Kush mountain range that Alexander the Great had once traversed. As the verdant vales of the northeast came into view so did our first of several stops. Small outposts of U.S. and Coalition forces comprised the bulk of our supply runs, but we were always offering extra services to our customers. Like an opportunistic taxi service, we would pick up anyone or anything that needed delivery within our planned route. That was how my view of the war and the world would change forever.

As we careened through the emerald passes of the Nangalam Valley, the sheer lushness and crisp clean air gave rise to desires for a simpler life connected to nature and her children. The U.S. outpost here was home to a small band of soldiers and contracted American teachers whose mission it was to establish a school for the area and provide much needed medical aid. The difficult task for us would be to put two of our helicopters in the crude landing zone. With a combined rotor distance of one hundred feet per helicopter, it would put us extremely close to the school, but this would not dissuade the children from inching as close as possible in hopes of receiving their anticipated treasure of candy or school supplies. On the ground safe and secure, the cargo would be deftly unloaded and passengers disembarked to be replaced by a fresh batch of the same. Being responsible for decisions on passengers and cargo, I sought out the camp coordinator to shop for standby personnel. His eyes brightened as he explained loudly under the rotor noise that he had a last minute change he was hoping we could handle.

"WHATCHA GOT?" I hollered.

"A little girl needs to get to Bagram for a spinal procedure," he said expectantly.

I had to lead him out from under the oppressive noise so I could get all the information I needed.

"Are you kidding me? You want to put a child on my bird during daylight and have us fly her through a possible shit storm?" I questioned.

"It's the only way! We can't risk a drive that will take days on these roads. Plus, she's safer with you guys!" he expressed passionately.

My heart sank at the prospect but I got back on the helicopter's internal communication system to let the pilots know what we were agreeing to. I knew the entire crew would have the same reservations, but how can you say "no" to a child? As I gave the coordinator the thumbs up and a beckoning wave he ran off so fast I thought he'd lose his boots. The passengers were repositioned to accommodate our new precious cargo.

The young Afghan was deftly carried onto the ramp of my helicopter by her father. Close behind was her uncle, clearly the two men were brothers for you could see the familial resemblance in the aquiline noses and the set of their brows. The girl most certainly took after her mother who must have the same stunning almond-shaped eyes. She was, by any standard, a most beautiful child. She was resplendent in her best, yet modest, attire which spoke of the love her father must have felt for her. Her long-sleeved blouse or tunic was a rich indigo with embroidered yellows, reds, and greens about the chest and neckline with matching trim on the wrists and bottom hem. The non-ornamented billowing slacks were perhaps the plainest item she wore. A pomegranate scarf completed the presentation giving her a look of innocence so that you could only feel protective of such a delicate flower.

With the loading of passengers and cargo complete, we rapidly departed the area so as not to linger and throw debris around the school as well as avoid becoming a target for a random rocket propelled grenade. As I stood behind my M-240 machine gun, I glanced back periodically to make sure our maneuvers were not frightening our guest. Leveling out at a higher altitude, I took a seat since we were out of weapons' range and could not help staring at her.

Having daughters of my own, I thought of how amazing it must be for a child her age to have a first helicopter ride—to see her country from the air and the sheer awesomeness of it. I motioned to her father that she could take a seat near my door so she could have an unobstructed view of the landscape, but he politely declined. I looked at her with her craned neck, eyes wide with a look of trepidation. My heart sank as I snapped out of my reverie and realized where we were. I was offering to put a child within arm's reach of a machine gun. And worse, I was offering to put her in the target zone of my door. We were flying in a war zone! A tear formed in the corner of my right eye and a huge weight began crushing my chest. I quickly put down the tinted visor of my flight helmet to hide the anguish and turned my head towards the door in hopes that the wind would blow away the stream of tears that I knew would give me away. The bulk of my body armor hid the heaving of my chest but just to make sure I stood and placed myself behind my weapon. Head slumped in shame, I drew several deep breaths and composed myself using my own scarf to wipe my face. *What was I thinking?*

The flight was without incident as we approached our home base. The helicopter was taxied into its designated parking position, and we went about the business of shutting it down, leaving our passengers and cargo inside until all the big pieces stopped moving and the noise makers were turned off. The look of appreciation on the father's face was enough to tell me that this was probably the most important event of his life. His daughter, lovingly nuzzled against his neck, arms wrapped around his shoulders, looked up at me with the brightest smile. She would remember this day for the rest of her life, and I was proud to have been a part of it. The simple act of delivering her to a place that would make it possible to walk again seemed no great feat to me. What I felt for my own daughters made it easy for me to understand how this father felt. He would have gone to any length to have given this opportunity to his child, and this country was full of fathers like him with children like mine.

The effects of combat are far-reaching and can impact for generations. How we leave this world for our children should represent the best in us, and if faced with a decision that will most definitely change their lives, we might do well to look at a child, putting ourselves in the place of their parent and ask ourselves, "How far would I go to protect this precious cargo?"

Believing Yoga
Poetry by Jasmin Serina

Yoga mat on the floor—
An open invitation
As I step into motion.

Busy thoughts,
Deadlines to beat—
Stress indeed.

Beginning in child's pose,
I reflect—
Perspective changes and gears shift.

Moving to a different posture
My balance shifted—
I wobbled and fell, for sure.

Continue with the flow
Surrendering how I feel that day—
I can do that asana, someday.

Concluding today's practice
The mind relaxes—
Breathing eases and stress decreases.

The good feeling of giving time to yourself—
Inner bliss is felt and
It is good for our health.

Goddess in Paradise
Nonfiction by Jennie Passero

When I travel, there is so much to see in the world that I rarely go back to the same place twice. Yet, there are a few places that lure me back. (And, I actually moved to one of them). One of those places is Nassau and Paradise Island in the Bahamas. Every time I visit I seem to connect with others and leave with a deeper understanding of humanity and myself.

My most recent trip was in January of 2017. My aunt was looking for a spiritual getaway, and I had been to the Sivananda Ashram on Paradise Island and thought it was the perfect place for her and me as well. Our initial plan was to take the daily yoga classes, swim in the ocean, and attend a three-day workshop about divine timing and synchronicity. As irony would have it, or divine timing, the workshop we were going to attend was cancelled. The only other workshop available was one about cultivating your inner divine goddess. As the Rolling Stones said, "You can't always get what you want, but if you try sometimes well you just might find, you get what you need." Cultivating my inner divine goddess was exactly what I needed.

This trip's theme ended up being about connecting deeper with other women and with myself. It was a beautiful experience but quite trying. All I have ever wanted was to be seen and understood for who I was. No masks, no hiding, just being vulnerable and honest. Even though this was what I wanted, I didn't realize how hard it was to let it happen. There was an initial fear associated with standing in my own power of who I was. It was funny how deep doubt can be ingrained all the way to the cellular level.

The workshop was held on a large wooden platform outside as the ocean air blew through and about twenty women sat in a circle. I was surrounded by women who were powerful and beautiful, and looking around this circle making eye contact with all these women created a palpable energy. I started to see more in these women than just what was tangible. Locking eyes with each individual woman felt like a camera that sharply catches its focal point, then everything in the background is hazy.

The workshop leader asked many questions which we answered and shared with the group. The one question that caught my attention was, "How would life be different if I believed the divine goddess worked through me?" The question made me realize how I still felt separate from the divine, how I still felt separate from myself. I could see it present in others but somehow it wasn't in me. But if the divine goddess flowed through me, I would have no fear of standing in my truth. All the self-doubt, criticizing, and giving my power away to others would slip away. It was a huge turning point for me. I had this moment of clarity and self-acceptance. This moment of feeling connected to myself and every person around me. To hear other women share their same stories and to hear other women share how they already honored themselves was refreshing. As these discussions continued, it felt satisfying to have these conversations with other women. To be honest without any repercussions or judgments and to feel supported.

One of the things I love about visiting the Ashram is the questions people ask one another. When we normally meet someone in our everyday lives, the first question we ask, after getting someone's name, is "What do you do?" This question bothers me so much. I have always felt we are so much more than our jobs. It is a surface level question; it is safe. It probably doesn't help either that I don't have an answer that most people understand. But at the Ashram, the first question asked, after we get someone's name, is "Why are you here?" It is such a simple question, yet it always has rich answers. Everyone at the Ashram is on a journey with an amazing story.

I remember one morning after breakfast I headed to the beach. I was wading in the water watching the cool waves roll over my thighs then pull the sand and small shells out from under my feet. A beautiful young woman was standing ten feet away doing the same exact thing as I. We made eye contact and smiled. She said, "I will do it if you do it." We both had been standing there for quite some time deciding when the ripe moment would be to duck under the surface of the waves but neither one of us had made a move. I let out a long sigh through a puckered lip smile and hesitantly said, "Okay." While the sun was sitting brightly in the sky, the ocean still had a chill to her, but we counted to three and both bobbed under the surface. I stayed under for a while to let my body adjust to the new temperature. I popped back up and the young woman was floating close to me.

We started with the "Ashram" introductions as we treaded water. Her name was Erin, and she was on escape from life. She visited the Ashram at least once a year because it replenished her body, mind, and soul. Right now her life was hectic, and she needed some quiet reflection time. The Ashram always offered that to her. She was a successful business woman who moved from New York to London. She was single, never married, and didn't have any children. She had spent her twenties traveling the world then she settled in London and started her own business. She could have fooled me. I thought she was in her twenties still, but she was in her forties. She had a youthful, gentle energy and a radiant smile and skin. She said she loved owning her own company, but it took so much of her energy. She wasn't able to travel and do all the things she loved like she had been able to in her twenties. She thought about selling her company so she could be freer, but she was afraid she had become too accustomed to the lifestyle she was living.

She shook her head with a smile on her face then asked about me. Why was I here at the Ashram? I told her this was my second visit here. This time I came with my aunt who needed an escape as well and wanted to have a spiritual getaway. At the time, I didn't call myself an Adventurer Explorer, so I always said I wasn't actively working because I had been afforded some opportunities that allowed me to take some time off. In actuality, and this applies now as well, my job is myself. My job is to rediscover myself, to take time to have fun with myself, and truly experience the joy in life. I normally didn't share much more than that, but there was a rapport with Erin. There was an ease to our conversation. My story began to unfold right there in the ocean. I told Erin that both my parents had passed away from cancer in 2014, six months apart from each other. While my parents didn't leave me with millions of dollars, I was still left enough money to be able to spend some time traveling, exploring, and following my whims.

Death is always an abrupt wake-up call to life. Watching two people pass away who wanted more time to live is unnerving. When they passed, my mom was sixty-one and my dad was sixty-five. I don't think

I ever took life for granted, but I think it is easy to get lulled into auto-pilot when cruising through life. And I don't want to miss the ride.

After I finished my story, Erin nodded voraciously understanding the need to not "just live," but to experience life. She was a fellow life traveler and appreciated others who shared that common interest.

There is power in connecting with another human being. Erin and I talked for thirty minutes in that ocean. We shared hopes, fears, joys and concerns; we were vulnerable; we were honest; we were our true selves. In that short time, Erin inspired me, and I was in awe. She had amazing experiences of traveling that she shared with me from spending time with monks in India to experiencing an intense Native American ceremony in Oregon. It made me crave traveling even more. To hear her story of how she started her own company and moved to another country, another continent, that alone elicited excitement in me for all the possibilities that life has to offer.

She was proof of what could happen when we take chances and risks and believe in ourselves.

I am the Artist's Canvas
Poetry by Arielle Witt-Foreman

I am the Artist's Canvas. Stark white and pure.
I am the Artist's Canvas. So much possibility I have in store.
I sit here waiting, patiently on her floor.
I know one day she will transform me into something more.

I am the Artist's Canvas. I watch her create masterpieces with ease.
I am the Artist's Canvas. I wonder if on me she will paint trees.
I have been waiting for a while. It creates trembling in my non-existent
knees.
I am perfect for her work. I do not understand why her glance flies by
me like a breeze.

The day has come! She has chosen me!
She looks at me for a while. I wonder what it is her mind can see.
She reaches for a paintbrush. She dips it in green.
I become excited to find out what my life will now mean.

I am the Artist's Canvas. She focuses on me for weeks!
I am the Artist's Canvas. My creator's love in brushstrokes speaks
Of release, healing, and cresting her emotional peaks.
Leveling herself out in paint, she finally describes herself as "meek."

Days and days pass and I wonder when she is going to end this feat.
Until finally, she places her brush down and exclaims, "Complete!"
She shouts, "This is my best work yet!" I am overjoyed! I cannot wait
to see!
I look down and do not understand what she means.

I do not see beauty. Only a dark, muddy mess.
What is she talking about? How can she call me her best?
Others agree, and I think they all need a good night's rest.
I start to win awards. What is this strange test?

Then one day in New York as I am on display,
Across from me a mirror they did lay.

I see myself complete for the first time,
And the beauty that I see could be considered a crime.

The muddy mess I saw when I first looked down
Was all that my perspective allowed, as it started at my crown.
I am a beautiful abstract
Full of color and a little black.

I resemble a Picasso! So vibrant with the Artist's soul!
I'm suddenly ashamed that I could not see that I am whole.
Now, I can fully see.
I am the Artist's Canvas. Beauty she created in me.

Mountain
Nonfiction by Amanda Rush

"It's okay to let me go," I whispered to her as we sat pinned to the side of the cliff. Panicked that each breath would be her last, she fought to regain her composure. She was still trying to draw strength and resolve from me, both of which I always supplied. Battling through was her way. We were battle buddies, she and I. Never one to give up, she always pushed the limits, no matter how far, even if it was to the breaking point. The competitive nature that fueled her filled me with desire. Yet, on that mountain, my grip on her slipped away with every breath taken. She was slowly coming to the conclusion that one of us wouldn't make it down from this place. She made her choice in the briefest of moments and was over the edge before I knew it. She visits me in dreams sometimes—an echo of a life that once was. I am forever changed.

I found myself stranded on the side of a mountain once. I sat there briefly in contemplation, wondering how I got myself into a mess such as this. It was *that* part of me that had fueled my desire to do it. I had that fire within to conquer obstacles and the competitive nature that had been my survival for as long as I could remember. As I sat there on a small ledge looking out over the Yosemite Valley, eight thousand feet below, I wondered if that would be the last sight I would ever see—if that day would be my last day. Perched there on my ledge, I reflected back, as those who are about to die often do, on a life well lived. What a waste of a good life to lose it at thirty-eight years old. Having come through so much trauma in recent years, to have it end this way was a shame, I thought. I had just started to figure things out.

I had been at war with myself for some time. Driven by my birth sign, my Virgo nature had always been one of striving for perfection in all things. I was extremely self-sufficient, practical, and driven to succeed. My old self was an athlete to the ultimate degree, and I dedicated my life to a sport that filled me with passion. The softball field was my battleground, and I was the conquering hero. Always the leader and always the anchor, I was looked to for advice, direction, and leadership. We always played to win. We lived by the motto to never give up and never surrender. We would come off the field of play bruised and bloody. Our bodies were broken and aching but were carried by the thrill of victory. Coming together afterward over meals of celebration and camaraderie, we bonded as a tribe and strengthened our resolve to conquer whatever came next.

That world was my safe place, the place where I retreated when life became too much to bear. When the realities of life threatened to darken my soul, I found solace in the world of my own making. I spent more and more time there to the detriment of my self as a whole, and I used it as my own drug to mask the horrors that awaited me in the real world. It was in those times that my best friend became that part of me that drove me to survive. That part of me whispered in my ear to push through the pain, the discomfort, the exhaustion, no matter the cost. All we had to do was survive, she and I. Survival was our ultimate goal.

And so, we continued, the two of us, for years and years in that way. Nothing else mattered. My need to succeed and her need to survive through any means necessary were all-important. When the physical pain from constantly running away from things got to be too much, we numbed the pain with alcohol and pushed through it. When the mental chatter telling us we were destroying our bodies became too loud, we drowned it out with music. When the insomnia came, we countered it with sleeping pills. Always running and always going. Sooner or later, you run out of places to run.

When I hit the wall, I hit it hard. The competitive part of me, the Ego, went silent. The will to survive left me. The darkness rolled into my existence like storm clouds across the horizon, so dark that I lost my way. Hope was all but lost to me in that chapter of my old life. No longer surviving, but merely existing in this world of my own making, my only choice was to let go.

I read an anonymous quote once that said, "Sometimes you just have to die a little inside in order to be reborn and rise again as a stronger and wiser version of you." You see this kind of letting go in nature, with caterpillars. Caterpillars come into the world as humble creatures, going on their way, and preparing for something that's just beyond their realm of knowledge. Driven by some force to prepare but not really knowing what they're preparing to do, the time finally comes for a period of stillness. The caterpillar builds its cocoon and when the time comes, it enters into this sacred space knowing on some level that reality, as it is presently, will be forever changed during this time of letting go. The caterpillar begins its transformation process by leaving behind the creature that it once was. Honoring the path that led it on its journey thus far and surrendering to the process of transformation, we all must die to self in order to make the transformation into a being that can fully express the beauty of our sacred and divine calling.

When the darkness came for me, I surrendered to it. It enveloped me fully and wholly, wrapped me tight and kept me warm. The transformation within occurred slowly at first. The ego that sustained me and the will to survive that fueled my purpose slowly released the grip from my existence, and all was still. I felt as though physical death would find its way to me in the coming months. I had already experienced emotional death, as well as spiritual death. My mental stability was beginning to waiver, and I knew that it wouldn't be long before I gave into its pleading to end the suffering once and for all. Then, when it seemed that all hope was lost with a crack in the darkness and a beam of radiant light breaking through, I found yoga.

Still surrounded in my cocoon of darkness, I began my yoga journey. I could see the path emerging with each new day. Day after day, I would go and learn to breathe again, learn how to move again, and learn how to feel again. Days turned into weeks, and weeks turned into months. My spirit was re-emerging, the light of my soul growing brighter. The crack in the darkness grew wider and wider as my wings began to grow. My soul's purpose slowly revealed itself as the process continued to unfold. Vision and purpose came into focus and with it, the transformation from merely existing, to surviving, to fully living.

My yoga practice eventually led me down a path to begin a nine month teacher training program. As I continued my study to become a yoga teacher, I was introduced to the guiding principles of yoga. Outlined in the *Yoga Sutras*, the eight-limbed path introduces a set of guiding principles in the form of the yamas and niyamas. As I pored over the text, I felt that tug begin that would later become the war between my old self and the self newly transformed from the cocoon of my old existence. The guiding principles seek to avoid such things as violence, lying, stealing, and possessiveness. Reading further, I understood that avoiding violence (ahimsa) includes one's deeds, words, and thoughts to oneself as well as others. As I read those words, I realized that my way of life before was fueled by self-harm in thought form as well as physical manifestation. My drive to be the best, to strive for perfection, and to win at all costs was causing harm. My broken body was a testament to the physical harm brought on by years of pushing through. My need for perfection was fueled by the false thought form that I was not good enough.

As my nine month journey through teacher training unfolded, I became more and more aware of the transformation that was occurring in every level of my existence. *The Bhagavad Gita* states, "Yoga is the journey of the Self, through the Self, to the Self." The process of yoga leads you down the path to your authentic self. It strips away, little by little, all of the illusion with which we surround ourselves. All of the protective walls we build up around ourselves are put into place in order to feed the illusion that we, at our core, are not good enough. Yoga is the reflection of ourselves in the mirror. The mirage we see in the mirror that has been created by the illusion of fear slowly fades away into the true image of ourselves as amazing creatures of ultimate beauty sustained by the most powerful force in the universe, unconditional love.

I began to understand that all my years of running from the trauma in my life was in vain. Avoidance is merely the mind's way of coping with things that are too much to bear. In reality, the trauma is already with you. There is no running from it because it is a part of you. You carry it with you no matter how fast you run. The longer you run, the heavier it gets. It stores itself in the body and throws it out of balance—mind, body, and spirit, it causes harm on every level. As this understanding washed over me, I realized that I could no longer carry the person that I once was. That person, that piece of me, was holding me back from who I was destined to become. A part of me knew the danger in that way of thinking. The negative voice would constantly say that it was the part of me where I drew my strength. It was the part of me that was the fighter, the survivor, and I would be nothing without that part.

As the battle continued, that part offered an alternative—that we could live peacefully together. I conceded for a time that it might work, the two parts of me existing as equals. However, as the months wore on, I realized that the old ways were slowly being replaced with new ways. That, as my transformation continued, old thought forms gave way to new. Things, that quickly brought anger and resentment before my transformation, offered understanding and compassion instead. Holding others in judgment turned into seeing things from their perspective and finding compromise.

I found myself on the side of the mountain, halfway through my nine months of teacher training. On vacation with friends in Yosemite National Park and after days of hiking, it was agreed upon that we would make the twenty mile round trip trek to the top of Half Dome, the most difficult and strenuous hike in the entire National Park. The night before the hike, I sat in my tent inspecting the state of my feet. All of the hiking we had done thus far had taken its toll, as blisters dotted the tattered landscape of my feet. There I sat in contemplation as to what to do. That old part of me that had grown silent over the passing months urged me to bandage them up and push on. Failure to complete the trip would be a sign of weakness. A few minutes later, as I hobbled around on my bloody and bandaged feet, I doubted that I would be able to even walk the next day. I made a deal with myself that if I could walk without pain the next morning, I would agree to go.

We were a mile in when the sun made its appearance that morning. Trekking at a steady pace, I stopped to take in the view as the sun warmed my face. Looking out into the vastness of the valley, I was overwhelmed by the sheer magnificence of the sights and sounds that surrounded me, yet feeling completely connected and one with the grandness of the experience. Our route took us up to the base of our first waterfall where we stopped to rest and restock our water supply. We continued on, climbing six hundred stone steps to the top of the waterfall and onward to the next one. Over the next few hours, we steadily climbed upwards towards our goal, passing through Little Yosemite Valley and making our way through a forest of Sequoia trees. By the time we reached the Subdome, we had gained four thousand feet in elevation. We were met at the base of the dome by a park ranger, for the rest of the way can only be accessed by permit. The last eight hundred feet of this hike is a combination of climbing stone stairs carved into the rock face and then climbing up a set of cables that have been bolted into the side of the mountain.

As the ranger asked for our permits, I took a moment to take stock of what I had accomplished and wondered if it was enough that I made it that far. I turned and looked at the path that I had just traveled and understood the accomplishment I had achieved in making it this far. I didn't need to go any further, but there was one last battle left to be fought. At the encouragement of my travel companions and that voice in my head saying, "We've come this far, don't quit now," I folded up my trekking poles, stowed them on my back, and stepped up onto the rock face. We slowly made our way step by step, to a series of switchbacks on the granite rock face. As we came to the end of the final switchback and stepped up and over the ledge, I realized that we had come to the end of the steps and the only way forward from there was climbing up an incline unaided and untethered. For the first time in my life, I was gripped with fear and unable to move. My friends urged me to continue. The voice in my head urged me to push through. Yet, I couldn't go any further. I turned around and sat down on the ledge, pushing myself back as far as I could and leaning back against the rock. I told my friends to go on and that I would wait for them to come back down.

There, I sat alone in the vastness of space. As the wind whipped and swirled, I looked out into the crystal blue sky and down to the treetops below. A truly exquisite sight. I sat there for a time, motionless. From time to time, hikers would come up over the ledge and continue past me on their way. As time continued to creep, panic began to set in. I knew the symptoms all too well. A tightness in the chest, shallow breathing, and the rush of blood as it drained out of my head, leaving behind the feeling of dizziness. As the panic grew, so did my realization that if I allowed the fear to control me, I would lose consciousness and fall to my death. I tapped into that old part of me that always pushed through anything and everything to survive. The idea came to me that I should make my way back down the way I had come, but in order to do that, I would have to lean back over the ledge that I was sitting on. The voice was there telling me that I could do it and to go for it. Each second, my breath grew more shallow and faster at the same time; on the verge of hyperventilating, my vision began to dim and numbness set in. In full surrender to this experience, I did the only thing I could do—breathe. A voice from somewhere deep inside said, "Just breathe." Yoga: The union of mind, body, and spirit through breath.

On that warm summer day as the wind swirled around me and the sun warmed my skin, I closed my eyes and lifted my face towards the heavens and took in air. I inhaled for a four count, held for four, exhaled for four, and held for four. I repeated the process over and over. With every breath, I surrendered more and more to the experience and let go of what no longer served me. In that moment, there was no doing, no forcing, and no surviving. In full surrender to that experience, with each breath, I let go of the fear. Using the tools I had been taught in my yoga journey, the journey to self, I guided myself back—back into a clear head space, back into my body, and back to living. Not too long after regaining my composure, two beautiful souls came down from above and asked if they could be of assistance. I, the person who would never ask for help, asked these two ladies if they wouldn't mind guiding me down from my perch. They positioned themselves, one in front and one behind and led me off the mountain to the solid ground below. I thanked them from the deepest depths of my soul, and they said it was no problem. Helping people was what they did every day. One was a trauma nurse, and the other was an EMT.

When my travel companions finally joined me at the base of the dome, we made our way back down the mountain and continued on with our vacation. My experience on that mountain stayed with me for a good long while. I thought about it daily. I dreamt about it almost every night for a month. Some would say that because it was a traumatic experience, it's only normal to dream about it. It ran deeper than that for me. I didn't understand it in that moment, but I felt like a piece of me was missing. I felt as if part of me, a big part of me, was still stranded up there, and that I had abandoned part of me and left it to dwell up there forever. I wondered if I would always feel this way because I had left something undone. Was it because I gave up before reaching the summit? I was only about five hundred feet shy of reaching the top. Was reaching the top and conquering that mountain the goal of that experience? Months later, I would ask my teacher for guidance. I asked her if in order to feel whole again, would I have to make the journey back up there and this time succeed in making it all the way to the top to retrieve that piece? As we sat there and discussed it, the answer finally came.

Tapas is the third niyama in the eight-limbed path. The fiery discipline brought forth to burn out impurities in order to, among other things, achieve enlightenment, find connection to the Divine, or achieve transformation. My experience on the mountain was a journey through the cleansing fire to shed what no longer served my highest good. In order to become who I'm destined to become, I had to let go of who I used to be. The trek up the mountain was grueling in every way possible—physically, mentally, emotionally, and spiritually. It tested me on every level. The fire within me burned hot and bright and in the moment of full self-discovery, it flashed as blazing hot as the sun and extinguished, leaving only what was true—my authentic self. There was no room for anything else. That person, who once was, is gone. I still think of her from time to time and, every once in a while, I dream of that place—the resting place of what used to be. Now, I set my sights forward and welcome what is to come.

One Piece at a Time
Poetry by Sophia Winters

Bring me your sadness,
Your heartbreak.
Let down your façade.

The smile,
The constant chatter,
The positivity.

Let it all fall away.

Don't hold back your tears.
They do not bother me.
Embrace the darkness.
Embrace it here with me.

I will stand by your side.
I will be with you,
Every step of the way,
Every piece of the journey.

I will not leave you.
I will not walk away from you.
I will not turn my back on you.

But, you must believe.

Believe in my power.
Believe in my ability to transform.

Allow me
To help you
Transform.

Work hard.
Give me every ounce of effort.

Pour out the tears from the heartbreak
That remains.
Blend the sweat with the tears,
So that you no longer know one from the other.

And together,
We will make it through.
You will be brighter, stronger.

Fierce.

One piece at a time,
You will find the warrior that lies within.

Stay with me,
For I will catch you.
Stay with me,
For I am your mat,
Your practice,
Your yoga journey.

My Yoga Mat
Nonfiction by Eva James

The first time I attended a yoga class after my husband's death I had been a widow for almost four years. I didn't really want to be on that mat. I felt uncomfortable, shy, and raw. Yet, I was so consumed by my grief that for the entire time of this widowhood I had worn only black clothes, which I was just going to replace with an even darker color, and so I was willing to give yoga a try. It promised to provide some of the healing that I so desperately needed, for myself, and for my then five and three-and-a-half year old sons.

The lights are dimmed. I place myself close to the back of the room next to a side wall, a spot where I feel safe in this unfamiliar territory, where I think I can hide and not be seen, as if I'm not even really there. The teacher, a lovely woman who opened the studio to find her own healing after her mother's death, guides us through a breathing exercise. As I'm lying on my rented mat, I'm thinking she picked this exercise and her words just for me. I'm starting to relax. She invites us to let go and breathe. I follow her prompts and feel my eyes filling with tears. I don't nearly feel comfortable enough to cry in public, not ready to answer any questions, not strong enough to let the stares bounce off of me, even too weak to receive compassionate hugs. So, I hold my breath and swallow the feelings that have risen to the surface. Once I feel calm enough, I go on with the exercise and switch from a short, shallow breath to a long and deep one. And with it the flood gates open, again. I bite my lips in an attempt to stop the tears that are already running down my face. I press myself onto the mat underneath me to gain control because, as soon as I let go, I simply melt into it. The more I relax my body and breathe freely, the more I dissolve into tears. That's when I realize, that for the past three years and nine months, I have been holding my breath!

I had to pull myself together and take care of my sons. I couldn't break down, not melt. I had to be strong, upright, to carry them through their young lives; I could not lie on the floor too weak to lift them up. It seemed like my breath would do that for me, make me go either way. If I allowed myself to breathe, I would crumble under the pain, drown in the tears. For the most part, I stopped breathing, unconsciously tensing my body to make it strong and firm, to weather this hell of a storm. I was in the paradox of chastising myself into near suffocation in order to survive.

The next time that I find myself on the mat, it's another four years later—a different state, a different studio, a different mat. This time it's my Yoga Mat. After sixty minutes of hot yoga (I specifically did not want to do hot yoga, and yet that's what I end up with!) I ask myself, "Why on earth did it take me so long?!" People kept recommending yoga to me, over and over, and I believed them as much as the books and articles I read about it. I wanted to go. It's just that I didn't. And now, still, I needed a tremendous kick in my butt. Ugh. This kick made me resist even more. I don't like to be told what to do, but who does? (You might want to remember that the next time you come up with yet another rule "for" your child. Or anybody, really). Yet, my essential self gave me that final push. It knew this push was in my best interest. I listened and followed the call to my Yoga Mat.

Again, the tears, but this time tears of joy. Again, the breath, but this time it makes me float.

I immediately feel like I belong. This is where I need to be right now. I have arrived.

Every time I enter this space, I feel safe and at home. It's like I'm under that protective, magical bubble they put around Hogwarts in the last of the Harry Potter movies to shield themselves from Voldemort. The only "cruelty" you come across here is a pose named after the Dark Lord. It's one of those that let me appreciate the fact that I happen to have found the perfect spot for my mat where I conveniently miss the mirror by about, hmmm, exactly an inch so I don't have to look at my grimacing face. Yes, my physical flexibility can definitely still benefit from a deeper practice.

"Come into seated, stretch out your legs into v-shape, biceps to ear, chest up, and now fold." The teacher says something along those lines. "Fold."

Fold? Pha ha. This is hilarious. My fold looks like this: arms down! There, that's it. That's my fold. Seriously. That's all I can do. For now, anyway. I know that it's possible. I see you do it, Miss A. But me, so far, the entire section above my hips, well, it's not folding.

"You can bring your chin to the mat if you want."

"If you *want?" Pha ha, I love this.* I'm still sitting here in a ninety, maybe eighty-five degree angle with no folding. There's definitely no chin to the mat, but I love it. I wish that I could already do it, but I'm fine with where I am right now. I can smile at my non-folding body. It cracks me up.

This is what's so beautiful here, at and on my Yoga Mat: There's no pressure. No competition. No expectations. It's not a race, and there are no comparisons. No striving for perfection. It's just me and my mat. Wherever I'm at and whatever I need in the moment, all that I receive are love and support. And, full acceptance! It's a safe place—a place of positive energies and healing.

My Yoga Mat holds me. It is soft and gives me a warm embrace. It is firm ground underneath my feet to help me stand in my own power. My tree takes root here and is able to grow, even transform. My eagle spreads its wings and takes flight. My dancer blooms into sensuality and grace. My boat's strong core takes me across the waves of life with integrity.

Here, in this undiscriminating and forgiving atmosphere, even my inner child feels welcome. The little girl in me, who so often gets left behind, I always bring her to my Yoga Mat, include her, see her, and honor her. My Yoga Mat fits us both. There is enough room for all of me in my entirety. I am whole. I am me.

My Yoga Mat is my island, housing my tribe. From here, my warrior goes on a voyage beyond the reef towards its north star. With my Yoga Mat, I gain balance. I breathe and my Goddess thrives! Namaste.

Enough
Poetry by Ariel Bowlin

Inhale, Plank.
Exhale, Chaturanga.
Inhale, Upward Facing Dog.
Exhale, Down Dog.
Step your right foot forward.
Step your left foot up.
Inhale, rise.
Exhale, hands to the heart.
Inhale to reach up and back.
Exhale to fold forward and down.
Flow and breathe.
Sweat and struggle through.

This ritual has been an anchor since I first started to practice Yoga.
It has grounded me through some challenging times,
Becoming therapy for my mind, body, and spirit.
When life is especially intense, I find myself dreaming
Of sun salutations, bounding away from sadness like a deer.

People have often asked me how I could keep doing Yoga
While struggling with a medical or financial crisis.
How could I care about movement and breath
When my life was in upheaval or I was buried deep under stress?
I am grateful that those situations have drawn me
Deeper into my practice.
Whatever the turmoil of the moment is, I face an obstacle every day
That is even more overwhelming.
It is the voice inside of me that fears the worst.
It says that I am not strong enough, good enough, or deserving
Of my dreams.
It says, *I can't.*
When I surrender to the rhythm of practice, I don't hear that voice.
When I reenact the cycle of life on my mat,
I become part of something bigger.

The framework of flow contains hundreds of possible combinations.
Yet, whatever transpires on my rectangle of foam, it always
Ends the same...

In death,
And rebirth—
A ceremonial cleansing of my self-doubt and expectations,
A calming of the constant demands from the monster within.
Each time I commit myself to my practice, I receive
A healing balm to my broken pieces,
So that they can knit together again,
Maybe even stronger than before.

The True Me through Yoga
Nonfiction by Michelle Petty

Yoga began for me in February 2013. I remember how nervous I was during the first class that I ever took. I like to be able to prepare for all things, and yoga was something that I thought there was no way that I could do. My cousin Anthea is a yoga instructor in Ohio, so who better to ask what to expect than her. I managed to take the encouragement that she offered, and I showed up for class.

It was a Hot 26 class. I was out of shape and new to yoga, especially hot yoga at that. I walked into the class and the studio owner, Trish, was there. I was the first one to class and she told me to just be, and whatever happened on my mat was just what was supposed to happen. I walked into the classroom; it was a large dimly-lit room. I liked this as I could disappear in the back where no one could see me. Trish brought me a strap and showed me how to get ready for class. By the end of the hour, I was ready for more. The reason I had come to yoga was for so much more than a workout.

In January of 2013, I delivered my stillborn baby, Olivia. My husband was overseas, and I had my little, two-year-old, Mason, at home with a friend. The depths of despair that I held in my body shook me so deeply that I thought there was no way out. *How could I ever come back from this?* I wondered. I needed to, though, for my family and most importantly, for myself.

I just needed something to help me process all of what my body had been through and certainly my mind would follow suit. I started therapy right away and was also on an antidepressant. I was out for whatever would help me heal instantly.

Then, I found my way to the yoga mat. At the beginning, somewhere in between, and especially at the end of practice, I wept. *How could a physical movement of my body cause this reaction? Was I normal? How could this be? What am I doing here? Maybe there is something to this? Would my healing evolve here?*

Through many more classes, I started to evolve myself. I cried a lot more, but I started finding physical strength as well. I was still going to my therapist as well as my yoga classes. I stayed on my antidepressant for six months, and then was cleared to stop taking it. I will always have some grief about the loss of my daughter, but a living grief that I can share with others to bring enlightenment and empathy.

I started taking different classes other than the Hot 26 classes that I was used to taking. I took a power flow class. This was new to me, and I liked it. Dripping sweat throughout class with steady movement, I was in love. I felt a real sense of accomplishment. I was so busy with the movement and the heat that my mind had no time to wonder. I was focused and strong. I was definitely drawn to this class and knew that I wanted more.

My husband was still deployed through this yoga journey that I was taking, and I still had my little two-year-old at home. I needed to be able to keep it together for all of us. I was able to do this through my two to three yoga classes a week. Then, one day at the studio, I saw a sign talking about a teacher training interest meeting. My husband had just returned home and he could see the difference in me. He knew that yoga was something that was now a part of me. He supported my interest and off I went.

A sister duo of yoga teacher trainers talked for an hour about what they had to offer. There were about twenty people at the interest meeting. I had no idea what they had to offer, but throughout the hour they talked about Baptiste Power Flow teacher training. I was drawn in immediately. I went home, discussed it with my husband, and then I signed up.

The training was intense and really opened me. I was raw and overwhelmed in the training, but it did offer me a side of myself that I did not know I could tap into. I was being prepared to teach yoga. I wondered, *oh my goodness, is this what I really wanted?* I learned a lot about myself and how to become a yoga teacher. I completed my training; I did well. I taught a few classes in the flow that was taught to me, and that was it.

By now, my husband and I were ready to try to have another baby. It had been a year since our loss, and we knew it was time. I was about two months pregnant at the end of my teacher training; a real blessing in my life.

During my pregnancy, I was closely monitored and I was not willing to take any chances. I was working full time and did not make time to teach any yoga classes. My personal practice stayed steady, and I am grateful that I had this to lean on during my pregnancy. I have learned so much more about yoga since the start of my yoga journey; even more so today. I was cleared by my high risk doctor in my pregnancy and had a healthy pregnancy. This was a very emotional pregnancy for me. A lot of grieving and gratitude occurred for me. I was able to hold space for myself, my new growing baby, and my lost little one, Olivia. I went on to have a healthy little boy, Julian. He was perfectly healthy and a real joy. So many tears were shed on my delivery day; tears of happiness from where we had come from and where we were in that moment. I know that our angel was with us and is part of our Julian.

Through the next year, I had no desires to teach a yoga class, only to take the classes. I was offered to teach a mommy and me yoga class, but I let my full time job and being a mommy and a wife mask my desires to teach, and I declined the offer. I thought about that opportunity a lot, and I knew that my true desires were to find my voice and stand in my own teaching power. I continued my own personal practice and shared my love for yoga with others. In my every day, I would find myself discussing asana with others or breathing and knew that I still had that teaching desire.

Another year went by, and it had now been three years. My personal practice started suffering, and I was not on my mat very often at all. It would be three to four months at a time between my practices. This was not okay with me, and I knew that I needed more. My parenting was suffering and the way I communicated with my husband was suffering. I felt out of control and needed grounding. I knew nothing in this moment except how to self-sabotage. What was in me was not present, and I let irrational thoughts of failure and "not enough" pour in.

I found my way to my mat one day in the studio and had a great class, so I bought a pass and started my regular practice again. I was back at the same place where I took my original teacher training. My fellow teacher trainer was now the studio owner and my teacher. I thought, *Wow, she did it and I did not.* One day after class, she approached me; I had been talking with her about my failures and she would always encourage me to keep my head up. She let me know that there was a therapeutic teacher training starting up and she thought that I would be perfect for it. This got me to thinking about the future, and I kept it to myself, but it was always on my mind.

After several more classes and a few more talks with her, I thought that it would be a great idea. My husband was deployed again during this time, and it was hard for this to make sense to him. I had already finished a teacher training and in his mind, nothing had ever come of it. I did not actively teach a class. Why would I start and finish another teacher training just to refuse to teach? I would have to find someone to watch my kids for three of the weekends while my husband was gone and neither one of us liked the thought of that. I would work all week, and then leave my kids with someone all weekend, just to start another work week. There were so many other issues that we came up with, but I still said, "Yes," to the process. My husband and I had issues through the beginning of the process, but we did talk about it. Later, I came to realize through the teacher training that I was mirroring my own self through my husband. This was a strong connection that we were able to have together. We were close enough to be able to have this deep connection, and I most definitely grew in this moment.

Through each yoga training weekend, a new revelation revealed itself. I was able to apply something to my own life. Maybe teaching would be something that I really was able to start doing. This thought both scared and excited me.

Yoga has evolved so much for me over the years. I now know that yoga is more than just the asana. Yoga is me every day. How I am in each moment. What I do for others and how I really hold space for myself and others as well. Holding the good and the bad in a peaceful place, letting whatever is to come next, come on its own and acknowledging whatever it is and sitting with that knowing—I can be present and rational. I do have moments where I let the shadows in and present the illusion of chaos, and it most certainly makes life messy in that moment. That is when I realize that I am not holding space for myself to see the good in the situation. I let stress do this to me, and I know that this will be something that I will need to continually work on. Knowing that I can always come back to my own breath, I fuel my body with just that.

Now, yoga to me is every day. What each day has to offer is an offering of life, and there is abundance in this. Everyone has their story and that is to be honored, but that is not what defines us for an entire life. I lost a child; this is painful and very sad. I can choose to live a painful and sad life by not fully experiencing what each day has to offer. I have taken many emotions that come with my child loss and have been able to share this and help with the healing of others. Knowing that I can hold space for another as they tell their stories and experiences, I know what it feels like to feel such tragic loss. This is also helpful to me in knowing that I can also be happy for others in their moments of joy. When I hear of someone else being pregnant and the joys that go along with pregnancy, sitting with this and fully having exalting excitement for them is more rewarding than I ever thought.

My future with yoga will be continual. Through my current teacher training, I have been introduced to many other avenues of yoga. I have found myself intrigued. I plan to tap into what I know to be true of myself—that I am capable of sharing my knowledge of yoga with others. Yoga is the everyday—breathing, holding space, and asana. I have just opened the tip of knowledge of what yoga has to offer. I have found a glorious yoga community around me, and I am so grateful for that. I know that I forever will have support in my journey in yoga and that support feels strong. I have discovered strength in myself and that also supports this structure.

I want to introduce yoga to kids and students somehow. This will be a journey that I know can make a difference, especially since I have kids myself (now six and three years old). I already see how they practice yoga on their own, and I want to be able to enhance this for them. Even if I only affect my own children, that will be a win for me. I want to see myself helping others to find their own strength and face fears knowing that there is always good on the other side. Knowing and sharing that with the bad is the good, and fears will be faced and will be overcome. This is huge for me and I know that it will take work, but I hope to reach the right people to help.

The world is full of yoga, and we don't always see it as that. People want happiness and health. We see that all of the time with New Year's resolutions and daily devotionals. Self-help books are flying off the shelves to meet the needs of the people. We are in a nation of instant gratification and if one could just see that there is gratification in the breath, then the rest will come.

Health and resiliency, stamina and strength—this is all harnessed in the breath. There is also bliss in religion, whichever religion boasts acceptance in your life. Living for a greater good and purpose to be a good person and live a life that reflects positivity can encourage others. I have found that living to be for more, and be more for you, elicits a certain super power that some may fear, including your own self.

I am so grateful for the journey that I have been on and will continue. I have always said that I am grateful for the military journey that I have been on as well. Married at eighteen, I moved away right after I turned nineteen, far away from home. So many times tragedy, deployment, emergencies all happened during my marriage. I am grateful for this military life we lead because it has taught me that I am capable of so much more than I could have ever imagined. I am strong and resilient. I have been on my own more than I ever thought, but I was never really alone. I can support myself, but I do it while married to my hero. I am me, my own self, but I am also me with my husband. He has shown me this life and we have lived it together. We have overcome and gotten stronger together.

I tap into this deeper, therapeutic yoga because I want to know how to be there for my husband more. By being there for him more, I am actually there for myself as well. I really view our marriage as coexistence together as one. I want to grow as he does as well, supporting each other on our path. I am grateful for the moves, the deployments, and our time together and apart. I am also grateful that I have tapped into a part of me that I may have never known existed. It is all in us—the power to do whatever we wish. Loving each other through it all, I truly believe that my husband and I are a unit.

Yoga has allowed me to see life differently, to be open to life and live in this world peacefully and happily. There is so much us around us, and I want to choose to live with vigor and excitement while being content in just being. Thank you, great big universe for the day, the light in the day and in the night.

Namaste.

Journey to Self
Poetry by Jessica Gibbs

I remember a time before yoga.
Before meditation and moon rituals.
Before stillness and peace. Before Self-love.
Life was filled with to-do lists and small talk.
Check. Check. Check. Next. Next. Next. More things, less love.
No room for dreams. No time to dive within.
A bit of me died each day in this life.

I remember when my practice began.
On a cheap, green mat in a snowy town.
The beginning of life breaking apart.
The end of a marriage. The start of me.
Mantras of self-love scribbled on mirrors.
Spoken each morning through teary green eyes.
Seated Meditation perched on a stool
Eyes closing as the sun dropped to shadows.
Pins and needles in my feet. Racing thoughts.
Emotions bubbling. Tears tracing my cheeks.
Distracted again. Avoiding myself.
Back to the breath. Inhale. Exhale. That's one.
Counting up to 10. Then, starting again.

I remember when I released my thoughts.
Gradually peeling layers of labels
Until I reached the center of myself.
When I met my own eyes in the mirror
Chanting, "I am enough" without crying.
When I felt a sense of peace bloom within
The confines of my ribs, my heart tender again.

Untitled
Nonfiction by Jen Villaluz

When physically you appear normal, how do you explain to others the constant state of pain you are experiencing? You really can't, so you suffer in silence hoping and praying you survive the day. Doctor appointments leave you questioning the diagnoses which don't give you any answers, only more questions. For a whole year, my days were fogged by prescriptions—muscle relaxers, pain killers, anti-inflammatory meds, and cortisone injections. Not being able to function without medication was not something I wanted. I stopped taking pills and turned to alternative medicine. Obsessing over natural remedies that claim to help or cure pain, I researched and tried them all to find relief. I finally realized that I wasn't living life. I was just surviving it.

On the verge of a breakdown, yoga found its way back into my life. We weren't strangers. We had history going back ten years. In 2014, I took my first yoga class in a studio with a live instructor and with other people in the room, and it was bad. Hard core hot yoga led to anxiety, and vomiting; it led to vowing never to do yoga again. Then a year later, yoga sought me out through a friend. When she mentioned yoga, I said, "Nope, not for me." She convinced me to give yoga another chance, ensuring me that it wouldn't be hot yoga and the class would be tailored for me.

Two years later and relatively pain free, I am finally living and thriving in my life. No, everything isn't rainbows and unicorns. Yoga teaches you how to find the rainbows and unicorns in every, and any, situation of your life. The most important thing yoga does is that it opens your heart and lets love inside, allowing you to love yourself, flaws and all. If you can't love yourself, how can you love others? For the first time in my adult life, I love myself and it's the greatest feeling.

One Day I Will Be Me
Poetry by Sheryl Hayes

Have you ever felt trapped inside of your skin?
Do you have a desire to be free, or to be someone new?
Knowing most of your energy and time are often spent
Living for someone other than you.
Lost in and on an obscured path
Of fulfilling roles and changing form
To satisfy everyone else at the end of the day.
Yes, you are empty and you still feel unborn.
Mantra: Today, I will breathe a breath for myself,
Take my first step to bounteous roads,
Where I can set goals and embrace who I am—
The person no one yet knows.
One day I will be me!

Renewing The Amazing Arielle
Nonfiction by Arielle Witt-Foreman

Since I was eleven years old, I've been given some type of medication to 'use' to deal with my issues. First, it was prescription medication, and by the time I was eighteen, I was using a self-prescribed cocktail of alcohol, prescription drugs, and illegal drugs in an attempt to calm my mind, body, and soul.

This continued until the birth of my daughter in 2013, when I found yoga, but I still struggled with alcohol. Alcohol turned me into an absolute monster. I always drank in excess and found myself having explosive outbursts in an attempt to release buried trauma. While some trauma was released, the manner in which I was releasing it created more. I practiced yoga here and there, but my practice was inconsistent. I craved connections with others but seemed to connect with those that brought out my worst instead of my best.

I entered a therapeutic yoga teacher training in February of 2017. Throughout my yoga teacher training, I still struggled with my addiction. I ended up connecting with a member of my circle who also struggled with her own addiction. We connected with the thought that we could support each other in our journeys to wellness and sobriety. She never wanted to officially commit to anything definitive when it came to ceasing substance use and continued to use, so I put my own healing on hold in an effort to connect with her on a deeper level. This was self-harm. This eventually caused me to subconsciously resort to deception, and lying ruined our connection. I realize that I had been operating from a place where I was giving away my worth and a part of me showed up to sabotage the connection in an attempt to save my own wellness. This gave clarity to me, and I found myself running for my yoga mat in the most literal way.

I spent weeks and weeks going to various yoga classes almost daily in an effort to 'use' yoga as a release for my trauma and tragedy in a healthy way. Prior to finding myself resorting to old ways in a new situation again, I had avoided going to classes in a yoga studio. Several of the reasons for this were shame, guilt, and anxiety about being around others. I feared being judged.

Before yoga teacher training, my yoga practice had been limited to short, fifteen or twenty minute practices that were focused on some sort of Instagram challenge. Whether it was my own challenge or someone else's, I discovered that I was doing yoga for someone else in the same way that I put my healing on hold for someone else. I made the decision to abstain from 'using' social media until I felt that I could once again connect with others in a healthy way. I completely made my yoga practice and teacher training about myself. That was the only way that I could even begin to heal.

The night that I made the decision to sever the connection to my friend in teacher training, my mala broke. I had purchased the mala at the beginning of the teacher training program. The next day, another mala broke. I collected the beads from both malas and placed them in a copper bowl for several days.

A total solar eclipse occurred on August 21, 2017, and I placed the beads and the bowl outside during the entirety of the celestial event. I practiced a few sun salutations under the safety of my porch during the eclipse and felt absolute calm. I had attended a few yoga classes in the days leading up to the eclipse, but I still left feeling shaky and irritated from either the detox I was experiencing or the residual anger I stored from previous situations or future anxieties. During the eclipse, however, I felt complete in each moment. I felt gratitude for being alive to witness such an amazing miracle in the universe. It was the first time in a very long time that I had felt such gratitude for my own life.

I have had moments in my life where I was not grateful for my life— when I felt like I didn't want to exist anymore. Most moments in my life were like this, even in the years after I found yoga. I was afraid of being truly open, I was broken in confronting those feelings, so I hid behind addiction because my mind didn't have the ability to stay in the present.

During the eclipse, I realized that I was in the present and appreciating where I was. I wanted to know more of this feeling, so I went to Yin and Flow Yoga class on the evening of the eclipse. During class that night, I felt the same grounding presence and peace that I found during the eclipse. After class, I found out that the teacher, who held the space that I was craving, also made malas.

I brought her the beads from my broken malas and she crafted a new mala and a couple of mala bracelets from the remaining beads. I found that after the mala and bracelets were completed, I liked the new creation much more than I did the two previous malas that had broken. In that moment, I was struck by a truth about things that break and are put back together—you need injury to know healing.

Throughout my yoga teacher training, I learned that attention to opposites brings healing in all types of trauma—especially brain trauma, moral injury, and post traumatic stress disorder. I have personally found healing by giving attention to opposites in asana practice and guided meditation practices. Through the practice of both, I realized that you have to know the darkest nights to appreciate the brightest days.

For years, I held onto my addictions because I was afraid to talk about them. Two broken malas taught me that I was meant to know the deepest pains because I am to know the greatest joys. I am to experience times of having no space held for me so that I can hold more space for others. As I let go of these pains and traumas and continue going to yoga, I find myself experiencing more and more peace in the present and discover that things are changing. I feel more confident. I am able to release my addictions and talk about my healing journey to others without shame for my past. Instead, I feel pride for seeking healing in the present. As I grow more in the present, my anxieties about the future dissipate. I see my life aligning in simple ways: A new job with benefits, a new healthy friendship with a beautiful soul who inspires my yoga teaching, deeper connections with existing healthy relationships, and, most importantly, I have a new confidence in teaching yoga to others. I am worthy to guide others on the mat because I am finally experiencing the healing of being on my mat.

I 'crave' yoga in the same way that I craved drugs or alcohol in the past. I've realized that I was really craving a way to experience the present and to escape from the feelings that dwelling on the past or future brought me. Those same feelings that I used to drown in substances, I am now confronting and releasing in the present moment as they arise.

Healing is a continual process which is why I always keep coming back to my mat even when it's not what I want to do in that exact moment. Within a few moments of stepping onto my mat and breathing myself into the present, I feel the urge to slip back into my old ways and I allow that urge to melt away. I forgive myself for who I was and welcome who I will be.

"The wound is where the light enters" *–Rumi*

How Yoga Found Me
Nonfiction by Jamie Henry

My yoga journey started this year in 2017, but my real yoga journey started about five years ago when I started to awaken. Yoga had been calling to me after suffering for years with depression and anxiety. I am a military spouse whose husband is gone more than he is home and I knew of no one who was a yogi or who took yoga; and doing physical activity at that time in my life was the least of my concerns. I was practically a single mom raising three young children. Two of them have special needs. Yoga seemed very minute at that time, but it kept calling to me from a distance, wanting to be heard.

Many, many years ago, I came across a website that offered free, in depth, yoga resources, and I spent all day printing them out with the goal of starting my own yoga practice. Life was so chaotic that it never happened, but I would find myself thinking about that booklet and how I wanted to start doing yoga. Time passed and life moved on. Another home, another city, and still there was no time for yoga. My heart was yearning for something deeper, yet my body and life said otherwise.

Something snapped in me one day when I realized my marriage was never going to become what I had always hoped it would be and that my relationship with my husband was a far cry from functional. Suddenly, my world got turned upside down and thoughts and feelings came rushing to me like a fast track of realization about my whole life in a brief moment. And the shy, small, invisible woman that I had become was trying to break free and grow. I was scared to death most days for even considering that something other than what I thought I knew was not really true. There was much resistance, and yoga screamed out to me even more! I lived no more than five minutes, on a good day, from a really great yoga studio. I would sign up for class and have to cancel because I couldn't afford to go, my husband canceled on me again, I was too tired, or the weather was crazy. You name it, and I had an excuse for it.

I was dealing with deep depression, loneliness, accepting the truth of my marriage and that I was a mother of three beautiful children who I felt incompetent as a mother to. My own mother's faults were slowly becoming my own. Yoga still cried out to me, but I told it that I was busy and didn't have time for its needs. Too many other people were begging for my attention and needed me. I started to become physically sick. And that's when things changed more for me, my diet, and reducing, to eventually eliminate, all of the medications I had been so easily prescribed. I actually started to feel better. I dropped thirty pounds in two months just from these changes. And, I got a little stronger, inside and out.

My awakening was still taking place with my view of the world quickly changing in front of me, and I began to remember who I was. I remembered experiences from my childhood and they had new meanings. I began to understand why my experiences in life happened. I began to understand that I was an empath, and I then realized why I felt so emotional over what seemed like the littlest things or why I was so affected by being around different types of people. I understood why I seemed to know the things I knew, even as a child although I had to keep this knowing to myself in order to stay safe.

Nonetheless, it was all coming back to me and more. I always yearned to be part of something bigger. I knew it was my purpose, yet didn't understand how I knew this. A long, long story later, I ended up in Clarksville, TN. An opportunity presented itself to me in the form of yoga teacher training right in my neighborhood. I was excited beyond explanation! After all of the years of hearing the call and researching different trainings around the U.S. and trying to find one close to me, I thought how awesome it was to have one right here in my backyard. I had to do it! It had to happen. I didn't know why, but it felt like my life depended on it. It turned out that it wasn't the right time for me as life's plan had something else in mind.

So, I waited and, in the meantime, I continued to grow and learn all I could cram into my mind until the opportunity presented itself again. I still did not practice yoga at this time. Crazy, I know! I finished my M.A. in Special Education and still didn't feel like I had a purpose. With my awakening still happening, in the midst of my husband's deployment, my marriage got turned upside down again; and although perfect for a brief moment in time, I still needed more.

It was then that I found the Priestess Path, the call of the Divine Feminine, on my heart. Once again, I was swept up in a whirlwind of unknowing and confusion while realizing that my mind and reality was still very, very small. I pressed on. I wanted to learn more. And through all the learning, clearing, healing, ritual, daily spiritual practice, and letting go, I was still missing something.

I walked into Yoga Mat. I had stayed small for so long thinking that I wasn't worthy of friendship and love and that I didn't belong anywhere, but at Yoga Mat, there were actually people who I could talk to and be around and they would get me. I started to attend some classes. I knew nothing at all about yoga except that I knew my soul wanted to do it. I finally did. Then, yoga training opened, and I took the plunge, made it happen, and hoped for the best.

Although challenging, yoga helped to open my eyes more and really see things for what they were. It also helped me to see that I am worth everything regardless if anyone else thinks so. During this process, I was still walking through Priestess, as it is a never-ending journey just like yoga. It helped me to see my higher purpose more clearly and allowed me to see that the only way to fulfill that purpose would be through yoga. Yoga was the missing link for me, and the reasons behind the why. Yoga is the deeper connection to the wisdom teachings, to the chakras, and to the divine connection through mind, body, and soul.

My yoga journey is very different than most, and for a different reason than most. It brings my body into alignment with the energy that exists around and within myself. It helps me understand the emotional abuses that I have experienced in my life and why I have struggled so much with it. And most importantly, yoga teaches me how to heal those wounds in order to move closer to the best version of myself.

Yoga has helped bring back my inner and outer power and taught me that it has been a part of me all along. I never needed to look outside myself. I was enough. I just needed to believe that. I have hurt and suffered enough. I can only control who I am and how I react to any given situation. I can no longer stay small for the sake of others. I must become the person that I was meant to become. Yoga has opened the door for that to become a reality. Although I am extremely nervous about what lies ahead, I believe I am ready.

As I came to the end of my training, many road blocks appeared in my life. Maybe it was the fear of failure or maybe all that I have overcome and fought up until that point was trying to give one last go in an attempt to keep me from succeeding. I have had levels of anxiety that did not make any sense, although the task at hand was not a difficult one. I have been through much more difficult and challenging situations in my life. There has been a major shift on all levels, but I understand where the shifts are coming from and why they are happening. Even through all of the emotions of fear, anxiety, and unworthiness, I continue to push through and refuse to allow them to conquer me.

Each one of us is a vessel of change. Alchemy at its finest resides within each one of us. In order to grow and become more conscious, which is what yoga asks of us, we must break down the walls that have contained and defined us, what we have been taught as individuals and as a society. Growth is painful. It always has been. History proves this. Science proves this. Higher consciousness thinking, which is what yoga offers us, is required to rise above our challenges and create lasting, and important, change.

These moments of challenge define who we are as beings, human beings. Moments where we have to decide if we are going to sink back into the norm or swim through the difficult currents to higher ground. These moments change our lives completely. They are tests of endurance and determination that each one of us has to overcome in our lives, time and time again. It is amazing the power the mind can have over us. The Maya that exists in each one of us and how vulnerable we become is quite profound.

My body has had a long, hard road, physically and mentally, my heart shattered many times, and my sanity questioned along the way, but yoga has helped put the pieces back together and make me whole once again. Yoga didn't give up on me when I didn't have time or love myself enough to try. Yoga will always be a part of my life and of my children's and for generations to come as long as each one of the awakened ones helps awaken others so that it can happen. Now that I am a High Priestess Initiate, I am able to understand even deeper the importance of transformation needed on this planet. Healing on all levels must take place, and yoga is a path to making us whole. Yoga asks you to stop and listen. To listen to your body. To listen to your mind and most importantly to listen to your soul. *What is it telling you?*

The reality is that we can call it what we may, but in the end all paths lead to love. Our world and each one of us need love, we need to be loved, and we need to remember that love is truly the answer. It is not about who is better than whom, who has more than whom, and even who knows more than whom. What matters is that you can love, be loved, and hold space for one another. I am you and you are me. Yoga can teach you how to love—to love yourself and others.

"You cannot extend to others that which you do not extend to yourself."~ Kelsy Timas

We must change the world, and we must be the change that we want to see in this world, as Mahatma Gandhi said.

Namaste.

Aho! And, so it is....

Crumbs
Poetry by Yvette Huber

I unroll my mat to knead myself into shape.
Hands and feet press into worn places.
Resistance melts with each gentle stretch.
Every morsel of movement, I savor.
My eyes rest upon a small hole in the mat:
A space opened through my practice.

Yet...I am filled by the end of Savasana.

When I pack up my mat,
Rubber crumbs spill to the floor.
I consider picking them up,
But choose to let them go.

Delving Deep into the Pit
Nonfiction by Sherry Ulansky

I've done a lot of crying on my yoga mat. Different kinds of crying—the slow trickle of one tear at a time, the sob that starts from your belly and shakes your entire body, and the full-blown water works and nose snot cascade. I was unprepared for the magnitude and depth of healing I was to experience by committing to time on my mat; hours of crying became a necessary part of my journey back to emotional and spiritual health.

I was born in August of 1960, six weeks after my mother graduated from high school. She had been a pregnant teen without a husband or the support of her family and friends. "Good girls" did not get pregnant in 1960. After graduation, she was bundled up and sent to the coast where she was to give birth and put me up for adoption.

Plans changed. She celebrated her eighteenth birthday, gave birth to me four days later, and married my father within a month. She returned home to the Okanagan Valley, a wife and mother, at the tender age of eighteen.

It sounds like the happy ending for which we all hope—a deliriously happy family unit of two loving parents and their adored and cherished baby daughter. Perhaps it was for my parents; I don't know. That is not what I experienced.

My childhood was challenging. Growing up with parents who had problems with addictions meant I didn't get to experience the comfort, security, and validation of emotionally-present parents. A big black hole formed early in my belly in response to the absence of expressed love and presence of abuse. It was a hole that would drive me to seek out other ways to comfort and validate myself, giving rise to my own struggles with addictions.

At five, I started to sneak my mother's prescription Valium and Fiorinal and take the occasional sip of the booze she kept hidden. As a small child, dependent upon my parents, it was the only way I could escape into oblivion for some respite from the craziness of my home. My mind began to devise solutions to my pain. Booze, prescription drugs, food, pot, nicotine, sex, and money all became the answer to my discomfort and the bottomless pit in my heart and soul.

I left home at fifteen and partied my way through high school, an Honours undergraduate degree and graduate school. If you know anything about 12-step programs, you could have described my life as "classically unmanageable"; the symptom of untreated alcoholism. And, it was completely out of control. It was imperative I use substances to avoid the continually expanding abyss in my belly. Leaving home, going to school, having the right boyfriend, or anything else I came up with did nothing to stop the all-consuming spiritual cancer I had growing inside. I was slowly, emotionally and spiritually, starving to death.

I believe we all have moments in our life when the fog lifts to provide a moment of clarity and the opportunity to assess our path. I experienced such a moment when I was twenty-seven. I was in grad school and had been partying with other grad students. I remember ordering two glasses of wine at Earl's and then woke up the next morning in my bed. What had happened in between that time was a blank. I realized that I had driven home in a blackout. That was enough insanity. Something needed to change.

My journey back from the brink of emotional and spiritual starvation started in 1987, with my decision to stop drinking and using drugs. Many things have helped me along the way, but it was my restorative yoga practice that took my recovery to an entirely different level. I began to experience what it was like to be "in my body" again.

One situation, when I was fifty-three, catapulted me solidly into my practice in reaction to a particularly painful healing opportunity. Thanksgiving dinner was finished and I was sitting talking with my mother and her sister (my aunt). I asked her if she was able to talk about the circumstances around my birth. I'd done an enormous amount of internal work, but there was something missing that I could not quite put my finger on. She said "yes," so my questions began. "Did you want me?"

"Yes."

"Did you love Dad when you married him?"

"Yes."

"What happened when you went back home to your parents' house a married woman with a baby daughter?"

Silence.

Finally, my aunt responded, "That is easy. Your mother was the town slut and you were the symbol of the family shame." Bingo! That explained the "feeling" of never truly being wanted I'd struggled with my entire life. The origins of the mantle of shame.

The crying started as I drove home—just one tear slowly trickling down my cheek. By the time I made it home, forty-five minutes later, the sobs were coming from my belly. It was Sunday night and I cried day and night for four days. I cried for the little baby and then the little girl who had been carrying the weight of the "family shame" for fifty-three years. Time to let it go.

Thursday was my private restorative yoga session with Tim. I arrived with my swollen eyes and red-streaked face and asked if he could witness something for me. "Of course," he replied. "Let's do some yoga and then I'll make some tea."

After the yoga was completed, I was sitting directly across from Tim drinking my tea. "Whenever you are ready, my dear, I'm ready to be your witness."

With my hands on my heart, I looked directly into his eyes. I called up the baby and little girls inside of me to join our circle and said, "My name is Sherry May Ulansky, and I was born on August 2nd, 1960. I claim my birthright to be loved and to love, to be safe and supported, and to be seen, heard, and honoured. I accept my path and commit to doing what I came to this life to do in service of all beings on the planet." The crying stopped and there was peace, tranquility, and calm.

The crying did not remain stopped, however. For weeks, I'd cry as I practiced my restorative yoga. Whether it was alone at home, in a private session, or at Tim's monthly Do Less mini workshop, the tears would come. My practice had provided the safe space for me to start to feel the pain, observe it, treat myself with compassion, and release it. I'd lived outside of my body for so long, I was unfamiliar with what it felt like to be in it. The gift of my restorative practice was that it allowed me to come back into my body slowly. I'd experienced much trauma in my life, so it was a necessity that my re-entry be gentle. A calm counter balance to the violent exit so many years ago.

One night, lying on the floor of The Path yoga studio, all warm and snuggly in blankets, it occurred to me that I'd finally let my guard down and was learning how to receive love, support, and care. Tim always treats us to a Thai head massage at his workshops. As I waited for mine, I realized how nurturing and healing it was to be in a studio I love, cocooned in blankets, waiting for the gentle touch of a head massage.

The tears had cleared a space in my psyche that had previously been occupied by the mantle of shame I'd assumed as a child. I now had a little more room to accept the things that fed me spiritually, emotionally, and physically. It is never too late to heal those deep longings and wounds. The baby and small children inside finally got to experience safety and nurturing.

As I finish this story, I've thought about how I'd like to say that I've had no reason for anymore deep crying on my mat. That I'd somehow made it to a place of enlightenment that no longer requires delving into the remnants of the black belly pit. Then, I realize I have both—the moments of enlightenment that are filled with profound joy, awe, and bewilderment followed by the cavernous grief, pain, and sorrow. Neither lasts forever; I know that now. As long as I continue to commit to my sacred mat time, I've learned that I never, ever need to go back to a state of spiritual or emotional starvation. I am eternally grateful for the impact that lesson has had on my ability to stay present in my life.

A wonderful friend and yogi talks about the importance of not trying to bulldoze down the internal structures and systems we've built to protect ourselves from our pain too quickly. My tears have slowly started to erode those structures away; the gentle clearing away of what no longer serves me. Restorative yoga calmed me down enough to allow that to happen.

Tears will always be welcome on my mat whether they are a slow trickle, deep sobs, or torrents of water. Without water we would not have rainbows. We would miss the magic of that moment when we look into the sky. I love rainbows, so I'll keep crying.

Namaste.

One Step at a Time
Nonfiction Guided Meditation by Sophia Winters

Stand on your mat in a relaxed position. Take a moment to transition from where you are today, from your daily life, and begin to focus on a place of moving meditation filled with gratitude, reflection, and awareness.

I love to practice at the beach in the morning, first thing, as the sun appears on the horizon and begins its daily ascent.

Close your eyes.

It's just before day break. Imagine stepping onto the boardwalk. Feel the texture of the cool boards beneath your feet as we gently rock from heel to toe on our mats. See the sand dunes covered with sea oats as we make our way across the boardwalk. Allow the first glimpse of the beach to leave you in awe of the beauty of Mother Nature. It is quiet and peaceful. There are no other people as far as the eye can see.

At the edge of the boardwalk, take a moment to stand tall and strong in mountain pose, grounded in this very moment. Inhale and exhale a couple of deep breaths of the salty air. Then, descend the stairs and relish the sensation of the powdery, white sand. As we slowly head toward the water, pedal out your feet on the mat. Think about creating footprints with every step. Feel each grain of sand.

At the water's edge, sit in easy pose. Feel the soft breeze ruffling through your hair. Stare into the horizon, searching for the sun. It is still hidden, and the blue sky is a blend of yellow, orange, and red where it meets the ocean. Begin to circle your torso in a clockwise motion, while focusing on the colors of the sky. Switch to a counter-clockwise motion. Look for the seagulls flying. Move onto your hands and knees for cat/cow. Lower your belly towards the sand and gaze up. Observe the cotton candy clouds high in the sky. Slowly lower your gaze and notice how the colors of the sky change. Arch your back and draw your navel to the pink sky. Repeat the cat/cow poses again, while imagining your body as part of the rising and setting of the sun. Shift into garland pose with hands to heart as you watch the sun peek out from the horizon. Continue to imagine your body as the sun and slowly rise up. Hands overhead and then outstretched. You are shining.

In warmth and gratitude, swan dive forward and run your fingers along the backs of your legs. Place your hands on the mat and then lift your head to a half-standing forward fold. Step back into high plank. Then, lower your body to the sand and roll your shoulders back. Come up into baby cobra. Move into down dog, keeping your heels off the sand. Now pedal out your feet. Crisscross your feet to the center of the mat and rise up into mountain. Shine like the sun and reach up high. Swan dive forward, and place your hands to the mat. Follow that with a flat back and then chaturanga to high plank, low plank, and baby cobra. Flow through another set of sun salutations at your own pace. Modify with one-legged chaturanga, pointing your toes to the colorful sky. Then, for the next set of sun salutations, come up to king cobra envisioning yourself as a mermaid, pulling up on the rock to look out over the water. See the glistening of the sun reflected on the water's surface.

On our last set of sun salutations, shift back into down dog and really stretch. Notice how your body feels looser, warmer, and more flexible. Hop to the front of your mat. Roll up and stand tall in mountain pose. Feel the sun warming your skin and the radiance entering your body. Allow the warmth to seep into your heart. Allow the brightness to push away the darkness. Focus on the energy moving through all the broken pieces of your heart, the light penetrating through the cracks. Your heart is glowing.

For the next segment, we will be walking down the beach to the pier. Let's take a little rest before we go. Move from mountain to chair pose. Then, squat down and roll onto the balls of your feet. Place your fingertips in the sand.

As we walk down the beach, be present in the moment. Acquire that presence by selecting pieces of the environment as focal points. Do you hear the crashing of the waves or the squawking of the seagulls? Maybe you hear the quiet of the early morning. What else do you hear? Use your senses to listen.

How have the colors in the sky changed since our arrival? Find the line where the sky meets the water. Do they blend together as the same beautiful blue? Out in the distance, the water is calm. As we bring in our gaze, the water changes to gentle swells and then comes rolling into the shore.

Notice where you are walking. Are your feet wet? Are you in the wet sand playing games with the surf? Maybe your yoga pants have even gotten wet because you miscalculated the crashing of the waves to the shore. Or, perhaps you have taken to the gentle slope where the sand is dry and the water no longer consistently reaches it. Consider whether your path corresponds to your approach to life—observer, doer, or somewhere in the middle.

Now let's stop for a round of warriors. Flow through the poses in your own way, at your own pace, with your own breath. You are your own warrior.

We'll come back together in mountain pose. Step your legs apart for wide-legged forward fold. While your gaze is down, look for shells. Most shells we find at the beach are broken. The whole ones are typically few and far between. Do you think the broken ones are any less beautiful? For me, I see art, even in the broken ones.

Rise up. Reposition your feet and move into goddess pose. Smile at the sun. Allow your smile to shine through your eyes.

Return to mountain pose. Then, pedal your feet for the last stretch of our walk. Stay with me.

We've arrived at the pier. Let's move into tree pose on the left side. Notice the beautiful symmetry of the pillars. Now, notice their strength. How often are we like the pillars, standing beautifully tall and strong while the world crashes in around us?

Transition to tree pose on the right side.

At the end of the pier, past the pillars, the waves no longer crash. There is only the gentle swell of the water. Where do we find peace and serenity without the constant crashing? We find it in on the mat, in our practices, in our surrender poses. King pigeon is my surrender pose.

From tree pose, swan dive forward and step back into down dog. Bring your left knee to your nose and then place your left foot down on the mat for lizard pose. Dip your left knee to the ground for a deeper stretch. Drop back into half split. Then, slide into monkey pose. Move your left leg into position for pigeon pose. Pull your arms to the back and puff out your chest. Begin to open your heart. Bring the back leg into mermaid. Finally, reach back around with one hand and then the other to find king pigeon.

In king pigeon, my heart is completely open. My head is tilted as far back as I can reach, sometimes even cradled in the arch of my foot. And while I'm there, the world goes black for a bit because I am so far inside.

Slowly release the foot and bring your forehead to the mat. Transition into down dog and repeat the same sequence on the right side. Notice what side you favor.

Let's take our last down dog and move into savasana. Settle into a comfortable position on the mat and close your eyes. Feel the steady rhythm of your breathing.

For the final part of today's practice, I invite you to surrender.

What does it mean to surrender? Where does surrender take us?

Think of a situation in your own life where you've felt overwhelmed, out of control, where you've wanted different reactions from the people involved. You have exerted as much effort as you can, and still you've been unable to find a solution or reach a certain outcome. This is the time to surrender. Today, right now, at this moment, because we're here. Here to reflect, to regain awareness, to focus and to realize there are things in our lives, people in our lives, situations in our lives that are beyond us. When we identify these feelings, these inadequacies, these insecurities, we are also able to recognize in ourselves our desire for things to be different. And when we recognize and express these emotions through yoga and meditation, we allow ourselves to grow. Because as long as we hold the emotions inside, as long as we keep trying to control them or ignore them, all that remains is frustration, heartbreak, heartache, anxiety, depression. But when we acknowledge our emotions, then we're able to let go just a tiny bit, to surrender, and move forward in the smallest way.

I'm not asking you to give up. I'm not asking you to lose that desire for a different outcome. I'm asking you to recognize that today the situation is not within your means, not within your control. I'm simply asking you to put it aside, for today.

Tomorrow you may decide to come back to it, to evaluate it again, and continue to try to make it different. But at this very moment, you are taking it out of your heart, releasing it into the water, down the path before you, between the pillars of the pier. It has been crashing into your body for too long. Allow yourself to find the peace and calmness at the end of the pier, knowing you no longer have to withstand the constant crashing of emotions, the endless churning and struggling. Let it go, let it go for today, for this practice. Surrender to where you are, who you are and above all else, know you are enough, as you are today, in this moment. You are strong, fearless, courageous, and brave enough to let go of the things that no longer serve you. You are able to push through the waters close to the pier and overcome the crashing.

Surrender, surrender to this mat, to this practice and find with your most open heart, the beauty, the serenity, and the calm that is waiting for you at the end of the pier. Believe. Let it go. Float in the water. Light and free.

Thorncraft

ABOUT THE CONTRIBUTORS

KELSY TIMAS is a Board-Certified Holistic Health Practitioner, Life Coach, and Wellness Educator assisting the world in discovering and recovering a life in balance. A lifelong yoga practitioner on a mission to serve humanity in their journey and return to holism, Kelsy invests her time and talents in people and organizations looking for wellness solutions that move us toward a more balanced and integrative world. Her vision for the future is the driving force behind the growth and development of her national Health and Wellness company, Guiding Wellness Institute Inc. Kelsy's drive and success can be attributed to her deep desire to help people create their best life, a natural entrepreneur and pioneering spirit that has never been afraid to create solutions needed in order to find "a better way", and the sincere belief that she is in service of her life's calling. When she is not teaching or working, Kelsy spends time with her family and close friends, living the message of "living well" she shares with the world. Devoted to her role as a military spouse, community service grows and sustains her need to serve those who serve and the families that sacrifice so much. She loves cooking from her home potager and taking time for regular sunshine and the outdoors. Her favorite people call her "naynay." Kelsy also enjoys reading, writing, pottery and house projects along with her deepest passion, yoga, meditation, and mindfulness.

ARIEL BOWLIN was born and raised in the Puget Sound area. She graduated from Western Washington University with a Bachelor's in Spanish and worked as a contract interpreter for the State of Washington for several years. She also taught Spanish Conversation at Everett Community College. Chronic injuries led her to practice and teach Yoga and Pilates. She now lives and teaches in Tucson where she loves to hike, read, and practice Yoga in the park. She is a breast cancer survivor. Find her on Instagram as @arielbowlin

About **E.W. DZIADON III:** Edward is the owner of Oakland Power Washing, father of four, and grandfather of one. He served as a Non-Commissioned Officer in the U.S. Army which allowed him to explore the vast cultures of the world. After retiring from the Army, he searched for a new adventure and found Yoga. His journey into the yogic world has been one of the most rewarding endeavors to date and has allowed him to connect with some amazing people. He recently completed a 200hr RYT training program through Guiding Wellness Institute and Yoga Mat yoga studio.

JESSICA GIBBS is an ATLien working as a pediatric physical therapist by day, and a yoga teacher, aerialist, and writer by night. She enjoys being outside, listening to music, writing, and taking adventures of all sorts. Her yoga journey began in December of 2013 and inspired her healing process. She now shares her love of yoga with everyone she meets and hopes to inspire others to practice kindness and love on a daily basis. You can find her and follow her adventures on Instagram under the name @gibby_smalls

SHERYL LIN HAYES, best known as Sheri, is employed as a Behavioral Health Educator, specific to the Autistic community. She graduated from Temple University of Philadelphia with an A.A. in Spec. Ed, B.A in Early Elementary, and a minor in Adult Organizational Development Communication. She is a literary award winner and author of many publications. Her first book, *If Life Was Made on Canvas*, was released in 2010. She enjoys writing both fiction and nonfiction, sometimes meshing the two. She's been writing poetry since she was twelve; finding poetry to be the bridge that joins language to her soul.

She first took an interest in yoga and holistic health to manage many of her own diagnoses. Successfully managing and curing many ailments encouraged her to grow in her practice and to help others with their own medical struggles. Yoga allows Sheri to weave together her many passions—exercise, health advocacy, literature, and visual arts, making healthy regimes pleasurable. Yoga has given Sheri a sense of belonging, discipline, and poise needed to work with special needs. When Sheri is not working or striking a pose, she is usually cooking it up, traveling, targeting her next photo shot or hanging out with her two children, husband, and her doggy, Bailey.

JAMIE HENRY: "I am many things; a military spouse, Momma to special needs children, and an RYT.

My love for Yoga started not that long ago. Yoga called out to me when I was at my worst and didn't know where to turn. I gave myself away to others. When there wasn't anything left of me, it was then that my awakening started. My world got turned upside down and I began to see everything from a different perspective; what I once thought was truth was not the case.

Along my journey of searching for the truth, I became a Life Coach, an energy practitioner, and now a therapeutic Yoga teacher. I also found the Priestess Process and the calling of the Divine Feminine. I am now a High Priestess Initiate learning how to continue to heal myself, as well as help heal the conscious collective in this world. Yoga was and is my missing link.

Through this long journey so far, I have learnt many things, but the most important thing of all is that I must nourish myself first before I can be something for someone else. My list of passions is long and continues to grow. My desire is to learn all that I can in life and in Yoga because Yoga is Life. Yoga allows us to connect to the Divine in each one of us. Namaste."

BRITTANY HOWARD is a receptionist at Southland Veterinary Hospital in Lexington, Kentucky. She graduated from Eastern Kentucky University with a B.A. in English and from Lexington Healing Arts Academy with a 200-hour Yoga Teacher Training Certification. This training enabled her to teach a series of sunrise yoga and aerial yoga classes that have helped inspire a lot of her nonfiction writing and general attitude towards life. In her spare time, she now enjoys a personal yoga practice, working on her writing, and spending time with her dog, Zoey. Find her on Instagram: @paws.across.ky and Twitter: @brittanylhoward

YVETTE HUBER practices and teaches at Yoga Mat studio in Clarksville. Tennessee. Her work on the mat will never be done.

A "Hello Kitty" diary sparked **LAURA HURN**'s passion for writing at age eight. By age twelve, Laura was writing book and science reports for fun, outside of her schoolwork, for her family to read—the makings of a Technical Writer. At age sixteen, Laura began exploring poetry and short fiction in high school and then through university.

Professionally, Laura's passion led her to become a Technical Writer and Communications Manager whose writing caters to a global audience. Currently exploring fiction and poetry again, Laura's writings are ever-inspired by her hiking and yoga adventures. And, of course Laura still journals, "Hello Kitty" diary (sadly) excluded.

Whether it's traveling the world, writing about her inner and outer journey, or grounding down on her yoga mat, **EVA JAMES** is always up for an adventure. She is very passionate about being a conscious mom to her two sons and empowering them to be their true selves. You can either find her somewhere by the ocean or at her Bavarian home, where she works on her vision of leading a peaceful and balanced life in hopes of sharing her findings with others.
Learn more about Eva at: www.findingmywave.com

NIKKI MARTIN is a writer and full time yoga teacher living on the east coast of Canada with her partner, Paul, and two playful kittens, Tris and Lu.

Her love of stories, both reading and creating them, started very young when she realized they could be both escape and salvation for a shy, sensitive and awkward kid who always felt a little bit out of place despite having friends and being very social. She drafted her first novel in grade nine and her first feature length screenplay not long after that, and has written many of both genres since. She hopes to share her work with readers over the coming years and to continue to share her passion for yoga while teaching and traveling.

She is an avid reader, a daydreamer, a movie lover, a sunset chaser, a stargazer, a love warrior, a tree hugger, a beach walker, a storyteller, and an ocean soul.

She was a contributor for *BreatheYourOMBalance: Writings about Yoga by Women* (Thorncraft, 2015). Her first novel, *A Momentary Darkness*, in the fictional series *Awake While Dreaming* will be available in 2018. Find Nikki on Instagram as @nikki_possibilities.

APRIL McDUNN: "My name is April McDunn, and I was raised in a small town in Virginia and currently live with my husband in Clarksville, Tennessee. I began my yoga journey in 2014 during the darkest time in my life. My knowledge of yoga was solely based on what I saw in books and online, so I was in complete shock when I stepped on a yoga mat for the first time. It changed my life. Yoga has been an amazing learning and self-growth path that I just could not keep to myself. I have a passion to share all that yoga is and therefore I became a teacher. I graduated as a therapeutic yoga instructor in October 2017 and have since been teaching at Yoga Mat in Clarksville. My goal as a teacher is to share the many ways one can live their yoga on and off the mat. I hope to show others that during the hardest of days, you still have yourself, you still have your breath, and you still have a yoga mat waiting for you."

JENNIE PASSERO: "I most identify as an adventurer-explorer, and I love collecting experiences. I feel like the world is mine, and I am hers. I have been writing for almost 30 years, and it is how I creatively express myself; it is a way for me to process my surroundings and experiences. Yoga is a way for my body to express itself creatively, but it sneakily found its way into my life.

Three years ago, I started practicing yoga because of my love for running. I was looking for a cross training activity that would enhance my running. I am not an advanced yogi, nor can I contort my body into amazing poses. However, yoga has been a "place" for my body, mind, and soul to align and reset. It allows me to access parts of myself that have shied away. It feels like something that belongs just to me. It has become a personal relationship between me and my practice. Something that started off as a necessity for my running has now become a necessity for my well-being."

Read more of Jennie's work on her blog at Amor Fati, The Soul-O Traveler here: https://jenniepassero.com/
Find her on Instagram as @thesoulotraveler

MICHELLE PETTY: "My name is Michelle Petty, and I finished my first RYT teacher training in 2014 in Baptiste Power flow yoga. I recently finished my therapeutic yoga teacher training in 2017. I have a love for yoga for my personal self and for others. I am married to a soldier and we were stationed here at Ft. Campbell in late 2011. We have two sons that keep us busy. My husband and I are originally from Ohio. I'm a dental hygienist by day and a yogi always!"

AMANDA RUSH is the co-owner of Yoga Mat yoga studio in Clarksville, TN. She gained her RYT-200 certification in October of 2016. Crediting yoga with saving lives, she has made it her life's mission to share her love of yoga and wellness to all who seek healing. She believes that we each have a responsibility, and the power to do good works in the world in our own way. Amanda splits her time between the yoga studio and her work as a government contractor with the U.S. Army. Recently retired after 35 years of being a competitive athlete, she is excited to be in a position to provide the opportunity for young athletes to find yoga at an early age. She is also honored to be able to provide a space for the veteran population to find healing through yoga as well. Amanda spends her free time traveling the world and exploring new places. She loves to be outdoors and finds her favorite meditation practice to be long hikes in the woods. She also finds comfort in the times when she can be by the ocean with her feet in the sand, and she is looking forward to exploring her new passion, kayaking! Her guiding principle is that we each have our own story, and that each of us is the hero of that story.

JASMIN SERINA is a registered nurse living in Tucson, Arizona. She was born and educated in the Philippines. She earned her Bachelor's degree in Business Administration, major Accounting, in her late teens. She finished her Bachelor's degree in Nursing soon afterward. Jaz migrated to the USA to pursue her nursing career. She had spent time as a health care volunteer in Cambodia and Philippines. She recently came back from Peru where she was a conservation volunteer. She was a contributor for *BreatheYourOMBalance*, Volume One. Her yoga journey has been inspired by her instructors, family, and friends. Find her on Instagram as @jazser4.

ERICKA SUHL is the creative nonfiction editor for April Gloaming Publishing and an adjunct instructor at Austin Peay State University. She received her MA in English from APSU where she won Dogwood Awards for creative and scholarly writing. She has published work with The Regenerates artist and writer's collective in Nashville, *Clarksville Living* (formerly *Clarksville Family Magazine*), and APSU's *Red Mud Review*. She hopes that her commitment to developing her writing projects grows to match the commitment she now gives to her yoga practice. She is also a fun-loving, if not disciplined, mother and dog owner. She currently lives in Clarksville, TN.

SHERRY ULANSKY is committed to lifelong learning and self-discovery. She has been a soil scientist, map producer, manager, and currently teaches advanced project management at colleges across Canada. She lives near Vancouver, British Columbia, with a couple of zany black cats who love to join her on the floor for yoga sessions. Her restorative yoga practice began in 2013, and it has led to new adventures that include kayaking with orcas and belly dancing. "The Magic of Restorative Yoga" and "Delving Deep Into the Pit" are her first published pieces.

JENNIFER VILLALUZ: Pacific Islander, mother, yogi, naturalist, and crafter, who enjoys yoga, the simple things in life, and time making memories with family and friends. "In the end, only three things matter: how much you loved, how gently you lived, and how gracefully you let go of things not meant for you."—Buddha

JENNIFER WILL has been a student of yoga since her college days in the early 1990s. She is a practicing massage therapist/bodyworker, yoga teacher, writer, gardener, cat-friend, and baker, among other things. Along with the occasional poem, she also writes nonfiction essays and fictional sci-fi/fantasy. More info about her massage therapy practice, Thai massage workshops, and yoga at www.earthdancehealingarts.com.

SOPHIA WINTERS enjoys walking on the beach, traveling, and jeeping, but yoga is her passion. She especially loves the tranquility and challenge of practicing on the water, and the paddleboard has quickly become her favorite weekend mat. This Cajun yogi is currently working on a venture, which combines her belief in the transforming power of yoga, along with her belief that yoga can be practiced anywhere at any level. Sophia is continually inspired by the IG yoga community in her daily practice and can be found there as @yogajourney015

ARIELLE WITT-FOREMAN is a yoga teacher, wife, mother, and essential oils enthusiast in Rockfish, North Carolina. Aside from spending time with 4-year-old Belle, Arielle enjoys painting and connecting with people about yoga and healing on all levels. After starting her 200-hour training with The Guiding Wellness Institute Inc. in Fayetteville, NC (@guiding_wellness on Instagram), Arielle's journey for personal healing took a drastic turn upward. Her journey and love for yoga healed her marriage and brought peace to a warrior who didn't know how to leave the battlefield. The blessings reaped from

BreatheYourOMBalance Volume 1 brought love, healing, and connection to her household. Arielle has continued to bring this passion and healing into her community, completing her 200-hour Therapeutic Yoga Teacher Training in February of 2018, and she continues to promote her passion of yoga and healing to everyone she meets. Arielle is also a student of Full Sail University majoring in Entertainment Business. She will graduate with her Bachelor's degree in September of 2018, and she plans to use her degree in addition to her yoga teacher certification to create wellness retreats for those affected by all types of trauma.

ERIKA WOLFE is co-owner of Yoga Mat yoga studio in Clarksville, TN. She received her E-RYT 200hr. designation in the winter of 2016. Her yoga journey began in September 2012, when she fell in love with yoga after that first class. Yoga became her new life. Yoga made the stress melt away. It helped her to find confidence, strength, and belief in Self. Curiosity and a thirst for knowledge led her further down this journey to Self, and to find the "magic" behind Yoga. Her definition of this magic is to be able to practice at a studio that is filled with love, kindness, and open hearts. And, that definition of that magic has become her life's mission. With the opening of her own studio, she is able to bring that magic to others. She is teaching others to let go of challenges, obstacles, worries, ego, and so much more—to just be in the present moment—using breath to move through asanas, becoming stronger in mind and spirit, and allowing the body to follow. On any given day, Erika can be found at Yoga Mat, greeting all that enter with a warm smile and a hug, teaching yogis how to hug the "correct" way, leaning toward the right so the two hearts touch. Believing that yoga is for Every Body, she has set out to bring yoga to every demographic within the community. She has spearheaded programs for veterans, children, the elderly, and so much more. Her vision is to bring therapeutic yoga to all who can benefit from it. Erika likes to spend her spare time grounding in nature. Whether it's hiking, kayaking, or sitting by the sea, she's always happiest when finding connection in the natural world.

ABOUT THE SERIES EDITORS

KITTY MADDEN is Thorncraft Publishing's Senior Editor. She not only edits every book multiple times as a line and content editor, she also helps with strategy and overall planning for the publishing company. Kitty is known as Thorncraft's literary midwife, bringing out the best writing from all of our authors. Kitty was once a professional proofreader, nanny, and substitute teacher. She is currently a Reiki Master, practicing in Clarksville, TN. She lives in sacred woods connected to ancient, petrified, coral-strewn streams. She practices continually singing healing tones, coaxing dancing waters from a Tibetan dragon bowl with Luna, a dependent, resplendent, transcending, ascending, canine Reiki Master.

SHANA THORNTON is the owner of Thorncraft Publishing, an independent publisher of literature in Clarksville, TN. She created the BreatheYourOMBalance brand and book concepts. Writing is her passion, and she is the author of two novels, *Poke Sallet Queen and the Family Medicine Wheel* (2015) and *Multiple Exposure* (2012). She is the co-author of the nonfiction self-help book, *Seasons of Balance: On Creativity and Mindfulness* (2016). Shana earned an M.A. with Honors in English from Austin Peay State University. She was the Editor-in-Chief of *Her Circle Ezine*, an online women's magazine featuring authors, artists, and activists. Shana is a registered yoga teacher with Yoga Alliance and earned her 200-hour therapeutic yoga certification from Guiding Wellness Institute, Inc. in 2017. Shana loves to be in the forest, running trails and practicing yoga. She teaches seasonal, outdoor yoga at Dunbar Cave State Natural Area.

BOOKS BY THORNCRAFT PUBLISHING

Nonfiction

BreatheYourOMBalance: Yoga and Healing, Volume Two, Introduced by Kelsy Timas, Founder and CEO of Guiding Wellness Institute, Inc. (Spring 2018). This second volume of nonfiction and poetry delves into the poignant journey of yoga as it heals, restores, and revitalizes life after life. Many of the contributors worked together in workshops and practices at Yoga Mat studio to infuse their work with not only the personal yoga journey, but the roots of the yoga community that connect us together as well.
ISBN-13: 978-0-9979687-2-9
Library of Congress Control Number: 2017959537

BreatheYourOMBalance: Writings about Yoga by Women, Volume One, Selected and introduced by S. Teague (October 2016). A collection of poetry, fiction, and nonfiction that focuses on breath and balance, this volume celebrates the life-changing practice of yoga. Thirty contributors share their experiences in this first collection.
ISBN-13: 978-0-9979687-0-5
Library of Congress Control Number: 2016953726

Seasons of Balance: On Creativity & Mindfulness by S. Teague and Shana Thornton (March 2016). Teague and Thornton co-write a book about creativity, meditations, affirmations, expressions of gratitude and mindfulness to help you through the seasons of life. Use this book as a creativity journal to inspire you and to prompt artistic creations.
ISBN-13: 978-0-9857947-9-8
Library of Congress Control Number: 2016931608

Fiction

Talking Underwater by Melissa Corliss DeLorenzo (August 2015). Authors have declared that this novel is a "literary gift" and that "book clubs will love this." Cattail, the adored beach near her coastal New England home, is Amy's place of refuge. When a mistake there ends tragically, almost destroying everything that Amy holds as sacred, she doesn't know how she'll continue, nor mend the rift with her sister that results. *Talking Underwater* explores the balance between the elation of

family summers at the ocean and the ways we navigate unbearable heartache to find new ways of being.
ISBN-13: 978-0-9857947-6-7
Library of Congress Control Number: 2015938787

Poke Sallet Queen & the Family Medicine Wheel by Shana Thornton (March 2015). When narrator Robin Ballard takes a writing course in college, she goes searching for her homeless father and wanders into the secret lives of her ancestors and relatives. Set in Nashville and the surrounding communities, this novel offers a glimpse into the superstitions and changes of a middle Tennessee family.
ISBN-13: 978-0-9857947-5-0
Library of Congress Control Number: 2015901106

The Mosquito Hours by Melissa Corliss DeLorenzo (April 2014). One turning-point summer places the grandmother, aunt, daughter, granddaughters, and great-grandchildren in the same home. An "OnPoint Radio" suggestion as "Best Summer Reads" 2014, *The Mosquito Hours* is a multi-generational story about how the women in a family attempt to keep secrets about their desires, spirituality, and motherhood. ISBN-13: 978-0-9857947-2-9
Library of Congress Control Number: 2013957635

Grace Among the Leavings by Beverly Fisher (August 2013). Hailed by award-winning author Barry Kitterman as "a deeply moving story, one not given to easy resolution," this historical novella is a child's perspective of the Civil War. Playwrights Kari Catton and Dennis Darling adapted the book for the stage. For information on bringing the stage play to your local theatre, contact us through our website. Visit thorncraftpublishing.com for upcoming performances.
ISBN-13: 978-0-9857947-3-6
Library of Congress Control Number: 2013938285

Multiple Exposure by Shana Thornton (August 2012). The "war on terror" has captured the lives of the U.S. military and their families for over ten years, and Ellen Masters' husband has been repeatedly deployed. In the process, she shares her desires to connect with people and to discover her own strength by training for a marathon.
ISBN-13: 978-0-615-65508-6
Library of Congress Control Number: 2012941646

Forthcoming

A Momentary Darkness by Nikki Martin (Fall 2018).
A Momentary Darkness explores the realm of fantasy by experimenting with the possibilities of alternate worlds and lives. For Kayla on Earth as well as Kale on Alpha Iridium, the two women must find their true purposes in life, while finding the courage to face the combative challenges around them. This is a story within stories that can be enjoyed by anyone who dares to wander in their dreamscape.
ISBN-13: 978-0-9979687-1-2
Library of Congress Control Number: 2017959704

The Adventures to Pawnassus by Shana Thornton and Brittany Brown (TBA 2018). A Children's book for the child explorer in all of us, journey with Luna & Salty on their Adventures to Pawnassus where they meet the literary dogs of their time and try to fulfill their dreams. After being abandoned, Luna finds a home close to Nashville, but her troubles are not over, and she needs the friendship of Salty, the Texas raccoon, to inspire a belief in the future.

For information about authors, books, upcoming reading events, new titles, and more, visit http://www.thorncraftpublishing.com

Like Thorncraft Publishing on Facebook. Find Thorncraft Publishing on Twitter as @ThorncraftBooks and on Instagram as @thorncraftpublishing

90008235R00083

Made in the USA
Lexington, KY
07 June 2018